DROP
THE
SKIRT

HOW MY DISABILITY BECAME MY SUPERPOWER

DROP
THE
SKIRT

HOW MY
DISABILITY
BECAME MY
SUPERPOWER

Amy Rivera

Amy Rivera & Associates,
St. Louis, Missouri

For information about permission to reproduce selections from this book, contact the publisher via AmyRivera.com/contact.

This book was edited, designed, laid out, proofread, and publicized by an Editwright team. Visit editwright.com for more Editwright works.

Developmental editing by Andrew Doty
Copy editing by Karen Tucker
Book design by Peggy Nehmen
Proofreading by Ruth E. Thaler-Carter
Published by Amy Rivera & Associates

Typeset in Garamond Premier Pro, Gotham, and Northwell Alt

ISBN: 978-1-7370008-0-8 (PAPERBACK) | 978-1-7370008-1-5 (E-BOOK)
Library of Congress Control Number: 2021907875
Library of Congress Cataloguing-in-Publication data available upon request.
First Printing: 2021
Printed in the United States

A portion of proceeds from sales of *Drop The Skirt* will be donated to the Ninjas Fighting Lymphedema Foundation. Visit WinOurFight.org to learn more.

Visit AmyRivera.com to request Amy for a speaking engagement or learn more about Amy's story.

Contents

CHAPTER 1:

Born This Way

As the doctor walked toward my parents holding their newborn wrapped up like a stuffed burrito, my mother could tell something wasn't right by the expression on his face. He had a forced smile and an unsettled crack in his voice as he said, "Congratulations." She dismissed the fear of something being wrong with her child as quickly as it popped into her head, thinking she was just overly tired and had the new-mommy jitters.

My mother gazed at her newborn, as any new parent would, but instead of being overwhelmed with joy, she saw something was wrong. The nurses stood in silence with looks of confusion on their faces as they desperately tried to process the situation without panicking my parents.

"What's wrong with my baby?" my mother questioned everyone as she searched their eyes for answers. "What's wrong with my baby?"

The doctor answered, diligently washing his hands with his back to my parents, "She is a little swollen from the way you carried her in the womb. It will go away in a couple of days, nothing to be worried about." He walked over and pulled the blanket back, revealing the entire right side of my little body. "She is just a little swollen, and it will all go away in a few days as things start to move. Like I said, nothing to be worried about. Congratulations." As any parent would, my mother clung to his words and trusted that the swelling would go down.

She couldn't have known—most doctors in 1981 didn't have a clue, as I would later discover—the swelling would "go down," but it would never go away until I found out what was really going on with my body. I'm two months old in the picture below. If you look close enough, you can see my little face was full of fluid.

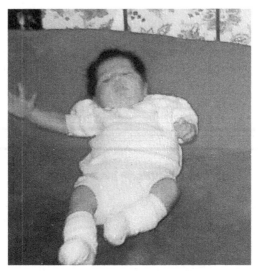

I am two months old in this
photograph, taken February 1981.

I tried to find a newborn picture of myself for this book, but to no avail. All I saw were pictures of me with a hospital blanket covering the right side of my body. (Only moments after my birth, the doctor had already begun a habit I would continue into adulthood: hiding my appearance from the world.) I was a bit confused about why my entire right side was covered and not just my right leg. I lived with a swollen leg my whole life, but the rest of my body wasn't swollen, so why was so much of my body covered by a blanket in these photos?

My mother told me that, when I was born, the whole right side of my body was twice the size of my left side. She said that I looked like two different infants, depending on what side you were viewing. The worst part of this was that she honestly thought she caused my swelling by the way she carried me in the womb. I'll give the doctor credit for one thing: Part of his guess was right. My swelling went down everywhere except in my leg.

We went to every doctor we could, from our family doctor to one specialist and then another specialist to another, all leaving us with zero answers. The medical field was unable to provide any diagnosis, treatment, or support. The burden of guilt weighed heavily on my mother's shoulders from the moment I entered this world.

As a parent, I can't imagine carrying the guilt of harming my child, even unintentionally. The psychological pain my mother went through was an ongoing nightmare for her. While my mother was going through her own mental anguish, I was trying to decipher what was wrong with me. I felt normal at home and around my family, but every time I went outside my home, I was quickly reminded just how different I was. The world wasn't kind to me. People stared and pointed at my leg as if I was some sideshow attraction. But why? What was wrong with my leg that people felt compelled to treat me differently? You can probably imagine how hard this was for me to understand as a child.

I recall the first warm day of spring in fourth grade. Everyone was excited to show off their new spring outfits! Everything was going well, but then it was time for P.E. I could feel my cheeks flush and my eyes well up as I worried about what the other kids would say about my leg.

I was standing against the wall waiting to be picked for kickball. I kept telling myself, *Any minute now, they are going to call my name,* as everyone else got picked for a team. Eventually, I was the last one standing.

The team leader shouted, "I don't want the girl with the big leg on our team. She can't kick a ball!"

I stood there feeling humiliated as tears ran down my face, and all my classmates started laughing and shouting, "Elephant leg!" It was evident there was a problem, but I couldn't understand why people were making fun of me. What made me so different? I never felt weird, fat, or gross, and yet I heard these things daily from my peers from that moment forward.

When I was at the zoo with my class, I found myself staring at the elephants, comparing my leg to theirs. I sat on the wooden bench, sobbing. That was the day I knew for a fact that something was wrong with me. Just as I was trying to gather myself, a group of girls walked by and laughed at me.

Shortly after that, the rumors started. One rumor that stays with me to this day was that my mother had sex with an elephant and that was why I was born with an elephant leg. Boys would stare, snicker, and whisper to one another as I would walk by in the hallway.

I wanted to be popular, but the few friends I had would only hang out with me in secret and barely speak to me at school. I once had a "friend" who would call me every day to talk to me about school. I tried to be a good friend and listen, but I finally asked her why she never talked to me in school. She changed the topic as I was midsentence. I soon realized that she wasn't a good friend. Years later, I ran into this "friend," and she confessed that she was embarrassed to be my friend at school and apologized for her behavior. It looks like there were two of us who dwelled in the past.

Middle school was not so different from the rest of society: My peers believed how your body looks determines who you are as a person. "Fat girls" are undesirable, less attractive, and stupid. "Skinny girls" are the opposite: desirable, pretty, and smart. And because I was different and didn't fit in with either crowd, like Belle from *Beauty and the Beast*, I was truly an outsider, and my feelings of loneliness resonated as painful echoes within me.

I was the girl no one wanted to be friends with. My life was a big puzzle with pieces that didn't fit the grooves. I didn't fit into the finished puzzle of life, leaving me feeling incomplete. This was a rough period of my life. I frequently skipped school and didn't eat. My leg hurt constantly. Some days I would stay in bed all day because it was too painful to move. My right leg felt heavy, and my hips ached the moment I stood up from my bed. Looking back, I realize I was depressed from the emotional and physical pain. I didn't know what to do or where to turn. I didn't even know what depression was! I was scared to leave the house, even with my family, out of fear that I would run into a classmate and they would make fun of me in public. It was bad enough that I was a prisoner in my own home, but nothing can describe the pain I felt being a prisoner in my own body, imprisoned by debilitating symptoms so constant they'd become a part of my everyday life.

What most people don't realize is that bullying echoes throughout a lifetime. You readily absorb others' voices as your own. I didn't know how to love myself in the way I should have. I only knew how to shame myself.

CHAPTER 2:

Standing Alone

By the time I started high school, I was officially known as the "girl with the big leg." The feeling of being different, combined with a swirl of anxiety, depression, and self-doubt, contributed to a downward spiral of questioning why I was here on Earth. Surely, God didn't want me to live like this. Why would he?

By 11th grade, I was facing a full-fledged identity crisis. Losing yourself isn't just painful; it can leave you vulnerable and willing to make poor choices to fit in. I integrated other people's beliefs into my own thought patterns about myself. Being a shy high school girl, I thought I needed to change the way my peers thought about me so I could fit in. I thought, *How could I do that?* After thinking about it, I came up with a solution for my problem: I was going to change my identity! I joke about this part of my life when I talk about it, but I honestly thought this was going to change everything.

I recall the day the thought of changing my identity became real for me. I was sitting on the living room couch watching *Saved by the Bell* reruns when a commercial came on. I normally hate commercials, but this one caught my attention immediately. Red and blue words flashed across the television screen: "Dreams do come true, and this is where they start!" My eyes were glued to the screen as my hand frantically rummaged through my backpack, grasping for a pen. I had my answer: I was going to enter the Miss American Coed Pageant!

I completely forgot about *Saved by the Bell* being on and ran into the kitchen toward the phone. I could hardly contain myself with excitement as I twirled the phone cord around my fingers, anxiously waiting for someone to pick up the other end.

Finally, I heard this sweet voice on the other end of the receiver: "Good afternoon, and thank you for calling American Coed." I was practically screaming as I gave the receptionist my information; she even commented on my overwhelming enthusiasm. As soon as I got off the phone, I ran into the living room to catch the end of *Saved by the Bell*.

I decided to keep this phone call a secret until I received the information in the mail. Every day for an entire week, I ran the half mile down my gravel driveway to check the mailbox. My mother was trying to figure out why I was so eager to get the mail every day. She thought I had a secret pen pal! Friday came, and I knew the envelope would be in the mailbox—but it was empty. I was becoming discouraged and thought that maybe this was a sign not to enter the pageant.

I held together pretty well until Saturday morning rolled around. I woke up with the pageant on my mind once again. As soon as the clock struck noon, I took off running as fast as I could down the driveway to the mailbox. I felt as if I couldn't run fast enough because my adrenaline was pumping. When I finally reached the mailbox, it felt like time had stopped. I couldn't believe it. There was a shiny red-and-blue envelope. I quickly grabbed the mail and ran up the driveway, tearing the envelope to shreds. You could have easily followed me back to the house by the colorful paper trail I left behind. As I read the words printed in bold black ink, "MISS

AMERICAN COED JUNIOR PAGEANT," I knew this was it! My life was going to change!

After running what felt like a marathon, I crossed the finish line into the kitchen. I stood there with a massive smile on my face, completely out of breath and excited at the same time. My mother stood there waiting for me to calm down so she could understand why I was so excited. As soon as I caught my breath, I said, "I want to be in this pageant," and handed her the envelope.

My mom didn't even look at the letter. She just said, "No way, Amy Jo." She would use my middle name whenever she was serious, which was my cue not to push the subject, but I didn't care this time.

I turned around and blurted out, "How are you going to tell me no when I'm not even finished telling you everything?" I walked away with tears in my eyes.

I sat in my room that entire Saturday thinking of a way to convince my mom to allow me to enter the pageant. Then it hit me: I would explain to my mom what it is like to be made fun of, and then she would understand and let me go!

I stomped down the stairs and straight into the kitchen and said, "You will never know what it is like to be me, nor do I expect you to, but what I do expect you to do is to support me. I will raise all the money myself. You'll see, and when I win that crown, you will regret saying no," and I walked away. Looking back, I realized I did not execute my plan very well. I never actually explained what it is like to be made fun of. My emotions simply took over. Welcome to being a teenager!

As a parent myself now, reflecting on this situation, I understand why my mom didn't want me to enter a pageant. She was trying to protect me from being hurt even more than I already was. My mother's excuse was that pageants are scams and the winners are already preselected.

Maybe she got tired of me pestering her, but she finally agreed to let me enter the pageant. It was time to show my mother that I could do it! I wasn't a salesperson by any means, but I had to sell this idea to people so they would sponsor me. I had to earn the funds for the pageant fee, the dress, makeup, and—of course—tickets, since my parents made it clear that they would not pay for this, saying it was a scam.

During school, I asked teachers, friends, siblings, and whoever would listen to my pitch. There wasn't a day I didn't ask for sponsorships. I was determined to reach my goal and participate in this pageant. This was the first time I was able to test my resilience. I went to every business in town asking for donations.

I lived in the small town of Hillsboro, Missouri, with a population of 1,675. We had two stoplights and one Hardee's. It took longer for me to build up the courage than it took to go around collecting donations.

Two weeks before the pageant, I was still 50 dollars short. My mom tried to convince me to back out and give everyone their money back. But at that time in my life, at that age, this pageant meant a new life for me, and I wasn't going to let 50 dollars get in the way of that. I went to a nearby shopping plaza and spent hours asking for donations.

By eight o'clock, I had reached my goal! I was so excited that I could barely sleep that night. I lay in bed thinking about what type of dress I was going to buy and rehearsing winning the crown over and over in my head until I fell asleep.

The next morning, I jolted out of bed, threw my hair up in a bun, and ran out of the house. I couldn't leave fast enough! I was excited to shop for my dress. Shopping was normally hard for me because my legs were different sizes. For example, I had to buy flare-legged jeans, which were *not* popular in 1999.

After finding the perfect pearl-white dress with gold-sequin trim, I had to find the ideal shoes. I needed shoes that were glamorous and stretchy! After four hours of searching, six stores, and countless tears, I finally found the shoes.

I had 13 days to practice walking, speaking, posing, and my speech in full dress rehearsal (wearing dress and shoes). I was completely tapped out of money and couldn't afford a coach, so I watched models on MTV and then practiced in the mirror. My poor sister had to be tired of being my audience, but she never complained. I became so focused on training myself that I would go to the music store in the mall and read all the fashion magazines, taking notes and then going home and practicing what I learned. Nowadays, it would be a much easier process, thanks to YouTube.

I was a bundle of nerves the night before the pageant. I paced up and down the hallway, rehearsing my speech until I couldn't keep my eyelids open any longer. I remember jumping out of bed at three in the morning, trying not to wake anyone up, but I couldn't help it—I was beyond excited. Boy, I wish I had that energy today!

We lived an hour away from where the pageant was, so we had to leave by six to register for the pageant by 7:30 that morning. My parents were not happy about getting up that early, but they were ready and out the door right on time. I was quiet the entire drive there. Nerves were setting in, and soon, the doubts started to creep in. I wanted to ask to turn around so badly but knew that was a bad idea after harassing my parents for months.

As we pulled into the parking lot, I noticed all the beautiful girls with their two or three cases of luggage. I knew I was out of my league. Maybe my mom was right. *Who am I to win this? I have zero experience, a swollen leg, and no makeup artist.* But I had no choice but to believe in myself. It was time to see how determined I really was.

After signing in, I had to go into the ballroom with the other contestants to receive our instructions, T-shirts, and the weekend agenda. When I saw the pageant outfit, I wanted to leave once again. We had to wear white shorts and white T-shirts with the red, white, and blue Miss American Coed logo.

I did *not* want to wear the shorts. I had my outfits planned for the entire pageant, and wearing shorts was not in the plan! What was I going to do? I recall standing in the long line of beautiful girls, thinking I didn't belong. I wasn't as pretty as them, and my only talent was having a big leg. I belonged in a circus, not a pageant. Within one hour of arrival, I wanted to leave twice. This was not a good sign.

As the line continued to get smaller and I was getting closer to the panel of judges for our meet and greet, my anxiety thickened as if there was pollen in the air, and I couldn't breathe. I felt a panic attack coming. I tried to play it cool, but the girl behind me noticed. She grabbed my hand and said, "You'll be great," and she softly smiled at me. We quickly became friends after that.

Rose was from the Philippines. She insisted I meet her family, who were at the pageant to support her. During my conversation with Rose's family, I was waiting for someone to ask me what happened to my leg, but that question never came. I wondered, *Is this what "normal" feels like? People asking how I am and nothing more?* I felt a little lost in simple conversation, to be honest. I wasn't sure what to talk about if I wasn't explaining why my leg was swollen. *What do people talk about?* I pondered on this question for a moment, then realized I could talk about anything I wanted, so I did just that. I asked one question after another about the Philippines. I was curious about her culture and was drawn to the kindness they were showing me.

This interaction with strangers was a pivotal moment in my life. My thoughts, cares, worries, and input mattered to them. This was the first time I had felt treated like a human being. I was ready to be in a pageant, not in a circus anymore.

After registration, we had to meet back in the ballroom at six in the evening in our new red, white, and blue shirts and white shorts for rehearsal. This was the first outfit we would be judged in. It was called Casual Wear: Miss Red, White & Blue. This was a group performance, and we had to dance to a pageant theme song. I can't remember the words to the song, but I remember those white shorts like it was yesterday! I wore the shorts with pride. Normally, I wouldn't, but because of my new friend Rose expressing an act of kindness that I had never experienced before, I was able to show myself the same act of kindness.

After a few hours of being in shorts, nobody had asked me what happened to my leg. I saw people looking at my leg but couldn't believe nobody questioned me. I have to admit, I was still unconsciously hiding behind people, chairs, and the stage when we were standing around mingling with others. I didn't even realize I was doing it until I caught myself. But by the end of day one, I didn't want to take my shorts off! I was finally comfortable in my own skin. For one weekend, I was able to embrace who I was, and it was empowering. I didn't want the night to end.

The second day arrived, and I was ready to shine bright like Sirius (the brightest star in the sky). I knew I had to walk with courage, confidence, and enthusiasm, and so I did. It was also a little easier with my second outfit. I had a green-and-purple dress on that changed colors in different lights. I picked this dress because I had an entire speech outline for it. It was supposed to represent me as a chameleon in the community. This outfit was for the Community Dedication category. The speech was the best part of the dress. I was going to KILL IT... and, well, I did, but not the way I expected to.

The contestants competed in four categories. During the Talent portion, contestants were judged on self-expression and entertainment. In the Community Dedication Presentation, contestants gave a speech and were judged on their answers to questions such as, "What is the importance of giving back to the community?" The third category was the Personal Introduction Interview, where contestants were judged on answers to questions like, "What direction do you see your life heading and why?" Last but not least was the Formal Wear event. This one was easy! All you had to do was look elegant and smile!

When it was time for my Community Dedication Presentation, I stood there in silence for what seemed like a lifetime, trying to remember the speech I wrote. Do you recall the dress that was supposed to resemble my personality for the speech I prepared for? Here is where I nailed it. I desperately looked in the crowd, searching for someone's face to focus on, then I took a deep breath, looked directly at the judges, and said, "I guess I wasn't meant to remember the speech that I prepared for you, so I'm going to tell you why I shouldn't be here." Before the judges could say anything, I started speaking from the heart.

"I'm different than most of you in the audience, on this stage, and you, the panel of judges. I'm different than anyone else in the world, and you probably have never met someone like me. I have a secret I would like to share with you. I'm sure you are questioning what I'm referring to, and I will show you as soon as I'm finished speaking. I avoid school at all costs, even if that means I fail. I avoid the mall, sports, or anything that deals with a social setting. Are you wondering what the heck I'm doing on this stage? Because *I'm* wondering what the heck I'm doing on this stage. I am beyond my comfort level, and, quite honestly, I'm struggling to stay on the stage, but I must stand strong and fight for what I want, and that is to be a girl who wants to be known as 'Amy,' not 'the girl with an elephant leg.' I took a deep breath and lifted my dress. See, I had a lot of practice at keeping my right leg hidden behind my left leg or standing a certain way so you couldn't really see the swelling in my right leg. When I had the white shorts on the day before, I had been able to stand behind other girls in the back row rather than right in front of the judges. I'm pretty sure they didn't notice my leg until now.

You could hear a pin drop in the crowd. I kept my eyes fixed on the judges so I could stay focused, but the tears started to fill my eyes, and the most beautiful sound came from the audience: a standing ovation.

After I wiped my tears and stepped back into my place in line, I felt Rose grab my hand and squeeze it. After the contestants gave their speeches, we stood there while the judges tallied up our scorecards. I was pretty sure I wasn't going to the next round unless I won a sympathy vote from the judges. I didn't expect it, but it happened: I went to the next round. I thought, *Well, at least I made it to this round, and that was a good run for me.* Do you see the problem here? I was already counting myself out of the next round, and in my mind, I had already lost because I had shared my story about my imperfection and you need to be "perfect" to win a pageant. I didn't feel perfect; I was happy to feel like "just Amy" for the first time in my life. My secret was out. Little did I know this at the time, but this was the first time I advocated for my disease and myself. There is power in vulnerability.

One at a time, each category winner was announced and escorted from the right side of the stage to the left side. I was on the right side of the stage along with the other contestants, a forced smile on my face. My cheeks were hurting, and I was becoming fatigued from standing on my right leg for an extended period. Maybe I wasn't cut out for this. I figured my mom was right: The pageant was rigged, and all the winners were preselected. As I was starting to accept defeat, they called my name to join the final four! I thought, *How in the world did I get into the final round?* I couldn't believe it. Looking back and looking at who I am now, I see why I deserved to be there. I have and always have had the eye of the tiger.

I stood there, silently gazing at the other contestants' calves, ankles, and shins, something I did when I thought about having a "normal" leg one day. Strange, I know, but it was my thing, I guess. Anyway, I was so focused on my thoughts that I missed the announcement of the winner. It took me a few seconds to process the fact that my name had been called. I quickly came out of the trance I was in and saw everyone clapping for me as it hit me: I won the crown!

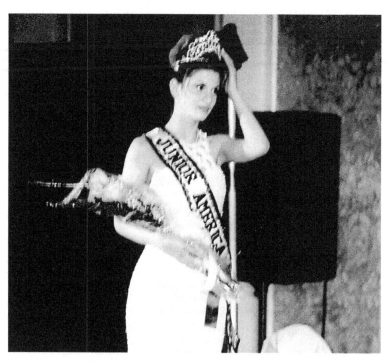

I wear the crown of Miss American Coed Junior Hostess, 1998.

As I stepped forward, I laid my eyes on my parents, who were reluctantly sitting in the crowd. I saw my mother's jaw drop and tears rushed down her cheeks. At that moment, it felt as if my life had changed forever. I thought returning home would be a more positive experience after winning the crown. It wasn't. Reality hit me after all the excitement died down and I was back home with the same group of peers in a small town where everyone knew everyone. I thought my new identity would fix all my problems, but when I arrived back home and earned the title "the beauty queen with the big leg," I realized nothing had changed. I found myself down again, thinking I was never going to fit in nor understand who I was—a lost life with no value other than a crown and a sash.

After a few days of crying and feeling sorry for myself, I decided to go volunteer at a nursing home close to my school. I thought if I was around others who had it worse than me, maybe I would learn how to be appreciative of my situation.

I volunteered for an entire year, learning about each resident. I spent countless hours with each of them and learned more than I expected. I realized that everyone had their own story and struggled with something at one point or another in their life. Volunteering there helped me find my purpose. I found happiness by helping others.

During my time at the nursing home, I remember seeing a picture of one of the residents in her early 20s wearing a nurse's cap. Her job was to organize the care for wounded soldiers during the Vietnam War. I was warned by the nursing home staff not to sit close to this resident because she had a habit of spitting on people. I saw this as a prime opportunity for a challenge: to see if I could build trust with her.

I saw the pain in her eyes and how lonely she looked. I couldn't help but relate with her and really felt like I needed to make a connection. I wanted to let her know she wasn't alone.

I sat on the other side of the table at the beginning of our visit. I approached her as if I was a patient and needed help with my leg. I gained her interest by pulling up my pant leg just enough for her to see. I saw her "nurse's cap" turn on immediately. She asked what happened to my leg, and that was the beginning of a bond that quickly grew between us.

I opened up to her, and she opened up to me. I sat with her for hours, talking about her job as a nurse and what I should do about my leg. As a matter of fact, I learned an interesting home remedy for cellulitis from her. If you coat the area of infection with Karo syrup and then wrap it with bandages, the syrup will draw the infection out! Luckily, I never had an infection, but I did ask a few of my friends in the medical field about this and they all agreed with her. This led me to understand she wasn't "crazy" but simply misunderstood. Someone just needed to take the time to treat her like a human being, like that Filipino family did for me the first day of the pageant. If I had judged her as quickly as others judged me, I would've missed out on this precious nugget life had presented me. I learned acceptance is tolerance and not to judge others based on appearances or physical tics.

I realize now that I am in the "disabled" category, but I refuse to be known only as a diagnosis. We disabled people are human beings with aspirations like everyone else. I was shocked to find out that I was one of 48 million people who suffer from some sort of disability, according to the 2016 Disability Statistics Annual Report. People living with disabilities face many different challenges that can negatively impact their quality of life.

Think about this for a moment: People like me who are born with a disability can't compare life to what it was like before we had our disability. It's different when someone lives a normal life and then some unfortunate incident occurs that impairs their quality of living. Both are unfortunate circumstances, but to me, it's a bit of an advantage to not know what life is like without a disability. It made it easier for me to accept my reality and make the best of it because it's all I've ever had. Your disability can be totally different from mine. Whatever your disability is, I encourage you to accept your reality and make the best of your situation like I did. Just because you won't be able to experience some of life's many great blessings because of your disability, enjoy and be grateful for what you can still experience. There's so much for us to be grateful for, and I find it so empowering to focus on those things.

People are used to thinking about disabilities in terms of the physical aspects but don't realize the emotional roller coaster we go through. Someone like myself, born with an abnormal swelling on one side of my body, has never known what it's like to be "normal." I learned to accept the fact that I'm not normal (whatever "normal" is) and adapt to what my life is. What other option is there? I can only imagine how difficult it would be if I had a healthy body and then developed secondary lymphedema as a result of an injury, infection, or cancer treatment. I sympathize. Both conditions are hard to understand and deal with, but again, I'd end up asking myself, *What other choice do I have?* I can't complain and be sad for the rest of my life. It wouldn't be fair to myself or those who care about me.

I've spoken to several people who were once healthy but became disabled after a tragic accident or illness. They explained that immediately after the onset of their injury or disease, they felt depressed, and a few expressed thoughts of suicide in the beginning. After a period, though, they adapted to their new life, adjusted their attitude toward disability, and started living again. I noticed some overcame the onset of depression with an overwhelming desire to accomplish goals even though they were disabled. That has stuck with me. Now, though I am technically still disabled, I live with tons of passion in my life by helping other disabled individuals find their superpower. I found mine!

I feel it is my purpose to use my superpower of helping others like me, and I owe it all to the mean old lady who spit on everybody.

Do you consider yourself disabled? Do you struggle with the same challenges? If so, let me leave you with this: Whether you were born with a disability or have experienced the onset of a disability, your mindset can and will affect how you perceive your disability. Perception is reality. How well you cope with the reality of living with a disability will determine your quality of life—especially your mental health. As Nick Vujicic would say, "Change your attitude, change your life."

Nick Vujicic was born without arms or legs. He grew up in Australia and, despite his disability, taught himself to do things like fishing and skateboarding. Today, he is a motivational speaker, best-selling author, and evangelist empowering people worldwide with his message. He's one of my all-time favorite motivators! The moment I would feel down about my situation, I would think of Nick and how far he has come. People like Nick gave me hope. Hope is a powerful tool, and I endeavor to give that tool to others.

CHAPTER 3:

Soul of Shame

Stop and think about how often you hear about how you can change your physical appearance. Every day of our lives, we are exposed to "suggestions" on social media, in magazines, and on TV about what our bodies should look like. I don't know about you, but I already had a negative self-image about my body, and these suggestions made it worse.

So often, people come across advertisements about how to get a "bikini body." These messages can seem normal; it's easy not to recognize the toxic subliminal message we are being told. It doesn't matter what shape you are in, the message is always that your body isn't good enough as it is. I do believe that every single person on the planet should try to eat good-quality, nutritional food to fuel their body so that it can properly function, help prevent health issues, and enable the person to live a healthy life physically and mentally. However, if you have a disease that prevents you from "looking normal," you should not let your mental health suffer like I did. Yes, of course, that is easier said than done, and as a young adult, I definitely struggled with this. It was freeing when I finally accepted the mindset that I was born this way, there is nothing I can do about it, and I have the right to be comfortable in my own skin.

Doing some research for this book, I was shocked when I found that statistics indicate that 94 percent of teenage girls have been body-shamed. However, body-shaming isn't exclusive to females. Teen boys and men are subjected to thoughtless opinions and hurtful comments as well. Nearly 65 percent of teen boys reported having been body-shamed.[1]

I was first exposed to body-shaming as a young teen. I was obsessed with the MTV dance show *The Grind*. In the show, they would try to make the women look thinner during the advertisements. This show was a hot topic in school. I noticed girls would dress more like the contestants or wear their hair like a certain dancer, and some would try to manipulate their walk to look thinner. I took note of the changes in their behavior because I always paid close attention to how others dressed and acted because I was so self-conscious about my appearance.

Most people have a definition of beauty. Some would say that beauty is in the eye of the beholder, but most define the standard of beauty by certain body dimensions, hair length or style, skin color, and type of clothing, based on whatever is in style at the time.

Our culture was preoccupied with "perfection," while I was just trying to figure out how to wear jeans! I had to stop watching that show! I shamed myself every time the show was over. We hear about people being body-shamed by others, but what if you are the one shaming yourself? I'm not sure which one is worse, body-shaming yourself or being body-shamed by others, but I will tell you, my experiences with body-shaming resulted in depression, anxiety, and

---

1   Larkin Lamarche, Brianne Ozimok, Kimberley L. Gammage, and Cameron Muir, "Men Respond Too: The Effects of a Social-Evaluative Body Image Threat on Shame and Cortisol in University Men," *American Journal of Men's Health*, 11, no. 6 (2017): 1791–1803, https://doi.org/10.1177/1557988317723406.

isolation. I couldn't go anywhere new and be around people who didn't already know me without extensive planning as to how I would hide my leg. I recall one time when five of my friends and I were going to a haunted house. We all piled in a van, and I made sure I sat in the back of the van so I would be the last one to get out. When we got to our destination, I purposely walked in the back of the pack. I literally planned out every detail ahead of time so I could hide my leg.

High school graduation was just around the corner. I was told, "Graduation is an exciting time. It marks both an ending and a beginning; it's warm memories of the past and big dreams for the future." This statement didn't feel true to me because I didn't have many warm memories of high school and didn't think much about my future. I didn't want to think about college, going to frat parties, or being part of a sorority because I knew I would never be accepted. I hated hearing, "You have to experience college life." I didn't like my high school experiences; how in the world could I think about a positive college experience?

I purposely skipped the "college experience" and floated around for a few years. All I knew was that I wanted to become a nurse so I could help people. I had known this from the first day I volunteered at the nursing home. The problem was that I didn't want to subject myself to what I had dealt with in high school by going to college to get the degree I needed.

After high school, I could only get home health aide jobs that paid minimum wage because of my lack of education. Struggling financially still wasn't enough to motivate me to push past my fears of rejection to get a degree. I wanted to leave this life behind and start a new one but didn't know how to do it. Without any guidance or direction on what to do with my life, I became complacent. I started binge-watching sitcoms for an escape every night after work.

This was a safe way for me to forget who I was. I was clearly on a dangerous road to nowhere.

I recall the day I realized I was damaging myself even further. As I was watching a popular sitcom one evening, I began to cry rather than laugh at the episode. There was a character who was overweight and was the center of several fat jokes. I realized this was the "norm" in our society. An overwhelming amount of insecurity took over me. This time, however, I thought to myself, *Why do I choose to continue to watch a show that's so negative for my psyche?* From that moment on, I stopped watching that show.

The next morning, I remember I was running late to work, and it was really cold. I got to work and was so frustrated with everything that I shared how I felt about not living up to my full potential with a coworker. As I was sipping my French vanilla coffee, she asked, "Why don't you do what makes you happy?" I didn't know the answer to that because I never really thought about what made me happy. I was always focused on what a miserable life I had. I sat on this question for a few months before I was able to find my answer. After thinking about it for some time, I couldn't recall myself being happier than the time when I volunteered at the nursing home. So, I decided to put in my two weeks' notice and enrolled in the nursing program at Rockhurst University.

I picked up a part-time job at the local hospital to gain more experience in the medical field. I wanted to help others feel better and care for them in a way I had never been cared for—with compassion. I was tired of being shackled to depression. I had to be okay with taking risks. Even if this endeavor failed, at least I tried. If I didn't try at all, I would never know if I could be happy. I was basing my happiness on my physical limitations rather than my actual capabilities.

This all was a big step for me in the right direction; however, I still had insecurity issues, especially when it came to shopping. Shopping could be traumatizing for me. I had a special technique for shopping to avoid being embarrassed. I couldn't tell any of my friends "I don't shop," because that would lead to questions. I came up with creative ways to shop without drawing attention to my leg. Anytime I went shopping, I needed to do some cognitive behavioral therapy the night before to prepare myself. When I would arrive at the store, I would wander around, picking out clothes to "try on" so my friends wouldn't question me. Then, we would all go into the dressing rooms and I would purposely pick the room the farthest from them so I could make the excuse that I couldn't hear them call my name into the hallway to show off the outfit. I would sit in the dressing room, looking at my watch and listening as they laughed at what they were wearing. I so badly wanted to be a part of that but just couldn't. After several minutes, I would come out and say, "I didn't like the way it fit." Then I would go back to the store floor.

Luckily, at this time in the early 2000s, long dresses and skirts were becoming fashionable, so if one would hide my leg just right, I would purchase it in every color. My friends would think I was on a shopping spree, so they never asked why I only bought dresses and long skirts. It was a win-win for everyone! I was good with putting a smile on and pretending to be happy, but I *hated* shopping and I *hated* wearing dresses and long skirts.

Between long skirts and scrub pants, I hid my secret and the chronic pain pretty well. Years had gone by, and before I knew it, I was in my late 20s with a leg twice as big as it had been when I graduated high school. I was great at pretending everything was okay until I got home. Every time I changed my clothes, I was reminded how miserable I was. It became too much for me to bear. It got to the point that I couldn't hide my leg anymore.

I was in so much pain every minute of every day and didn't know what to do. I felt pain from the moment my feet hit the floor in the mornings. I had neuropathy from the severe swelling in my right leg. My feet felt like tiny needles were puncturing my skin when I stood up. The pain radiated from my feet to my hips, back, and overall lower body. My entire body ached as if I had arthritis. My left knee would give out or freeze up from the overcompensation. I couldn't bend my right leg when I walked; instead, I would swing my right leg with momentum so I could carry that extra weight around. This was obviously hard on my skeletal structure.

I didn't know what else to do, so I started to drink the pain away and take painkillers. I didn't see a hopeful future in pain management. I would go out all the time with my girlfriends and drink the night away, seeking to numb the pain. This obviously didn't help my leg at all. It actually made the pain much worse and exasperated my swelling—and the headache the next day was terrible.

In 2003, I met someone new, and I was dreading telling him about my leg. This wasn't my first time dating, but it was the first time I was afraid someone would leave me because of my leg.

I'd had two serious relationships before. My first real relationship was in high school. He was a gentleman about my leg, and believe it or not, we are still friends to this day. The second relationship I was in was a little different. It was toxic from the start, but I told myself I was lucky to even have him with a body like mine. He often said I was getting fat in certain areas and that I needed to try harder to lose weight, so I dropped my calorie intake to 500 to 700 calories a day. What I didn't know was my leg was beginning to swell to the point the fluid was backing up into my abdominal and pelvic areas, causing me to look "fluffy." Needless to say, I was traumatized by the idea of telling this new love interest about my leg.

When we first started talking, I didn't say anything about it. I wasn't sure what I was going to say or how I was going to bring it up, so I tried to forget about it. After a few days of talking, I finally broke the news to him. I said, "Please don't laugh. You can leave, but just be nice about it." I showed him my leg and said what everyone else said: "It's just swelling for no reason."

He didn't seem surprised. He sat quietly for a few seconds and then said, "I don't care about that." We got married that same year.

The late-night barhopping didn't stop after marriage. It got worse. I had married a marine who was an alcoholic. We spent several nights out at the bars with his fellow marines and their wives. This was not only toxic for my body but for my marriage as well. I soon had more than just swelling problems. I had marital problems. It felt like the more my leg would swell, the more he would stay out drinking, so rather than stay home alone, I went with him.

The problem with turning to alcohol to numb the pain was that once I sobered up, my problems were still there. Not only were they still there, but they were much worse. Drinking made my lymphedema so much worse that eventually I had to give up my nursing career. My leg was so big that I couldn't wear pants anymore. It looked like a tree trunk, and I couldn't stand for very long. The 12-hour shifts were too taxing on me, causing my leg to swell even more.

Once again, I was lost. I was downright miserable! I hated the thing that was attached to my body, and I hated my life. What was I to do? I started numbing myself constantly by binge-drinking. I would have one or two Bloody Marys, a shot of tequila, and vodka with lime every night and stagger into the shower, vomiting as I washed my hair to get ready for work. This wasn't a flattering time of my life. As I continued to drink my pain away, my leg became even worse, my husband was now cheating on me, and I was on a hamster wheel with no way out.

My husband got out of the military, and we moved to St. Louis (my hometown) from Kansas City (where we had been stationed) in a desperate attempt to save our marriage. My life was going nowhere, and I now had two children to look after—my daughter and my niece, whom I'd adopted. I couldn't throw in the towel if I wanted to. One day, I asked myself, *What am I supposed to be doing with my life? Why do I have this thing attached to my body? There has to be a reason!*

I finally hit a brick wall in 2007. I decided to go back to school and get another degree so I could go back to helping people. That was the only thing that made my heart happy while distracting me from my physical pain and depression. I enrolled in an online course, and four years later, I received a bachelor's degree in business management. I wanted to be a hospital administrator. I thought that would allow me to stay in the medical field and have a job that wasn't on my feet all the time.

After getting my degree, I created a résumé and put it out there to see what I could get. A well-known retirement and long-term care company in St. Louis reached out to me for an interview. I was excited, even though it wasn't a hospital administrator position, because I was still going to be in the medical field helping people!

Things started off well, and after a month, I got promoted to the corporate office. I had never worked in an office environment before, so this was new territory for me. Of course, one of the first things that came to mind was that I had to make sure I had enough skirts to rotate through. Luckily, I had plenty.

Life was turning out to be great! My husband and I got through our rocky patch (or so I thought), the kids were doing great in school, we bought our first home, and I was making great money. After much thought, we decided to have a baby. This would be the second pregnancy for my body to carry. At first, I had several reservations. The main one was my age. I wasn't as young as I had been with my first child.

I had my daughter, Jade, at the age of 20 during my second relationship. The only complication I had with that pregnancy was my leg swelling even more. I figured it was general pregnancy swelling and it would go back down after I had my daughter, and it did, for the most part.

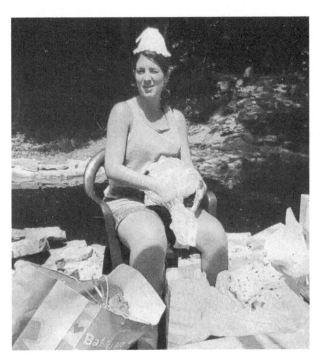

My first baby shower, 1999.

This time, I was in my mid-30s, and my leg was the worst it had ever been. Even with that being said, we didn't know how dangerous a pregnancy would be for me. I was considered a high-risk pregnancy because of my leg, so I had twice as many doctor appointments as normal.

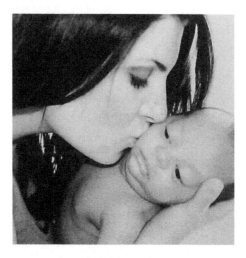

My second child was born in 2012.

As I got further along in my pregnancy, my leg became worse. I ended up having my son seven weeks early. The pressure of the baby was cutting the circulation off from my leg to the point it was turning black, and I had to go in for an emergency C-section in mid-March 2012. I knew that after this pregnancy, I couldn't have any more children.

After seven weeks of maternity leave, I went back to work. It was hard leaving my son, knowing he was premature, but I had bills to pay. I enjoyed my job, but something was missing, and I couldn't help thinking there was more I was meant for. I wasn't helping people the way I wanted to. I knew deep down in my heart I wanted to make a difference in the world. That tugged on me a little bit, but for the first time in my life, I felt empowered by the income I was making. I felt good about myself because I wasn't struggling making minimum wage, so I stuck around in the job.

Coworkers never asked me why I wore dresses; they just told me that I looked great in them! That made it easy for me to continue to hide the painful secret I kept underneath my skirt.

I had started working in the corporate office in October, and after several months, summer came, and oh, how the summer breeze inspires you to be free and careless. I loved the summer, even though I never felt comfortable enough to fully enjoy it. I lived in a subdivision that had a community pool, and every summer, I would walk down to the pool with my family and friends. Like anyone else, I had to prepare for a day at the pool, but it was a little different for me. Not only did I need to think about packing sunscreen, towels, and hats, I also had to pick out a swimsuit cover that was long enough to cover my leg, I needed closed-toe water shoes that looked like they belonged at the beach, then I had to have two towels: one for me to lie on and the other to cover my leg from the sun. I'm telling you, I had a plan for everything—except for being open about my leg.

For someone who planned meticulously for everything, I didn't plan for what was about to happen next. I was sitting at my desk talking with a coworker about summer plans. I don't recall the exact conversation, but I ended up asking her if she would like to come over and go swimming. As soon as it came out of my mouth, I wanted to retract my question, but unfortunately, it isn't like an email you can "unsend" before the recipient opens it. If she said yes, my secret would be out! I was terrified she would ask me questions about my leg once she saw it. As I was having this freak-out session in my head, she answered me.

I wasn't sure if I heard her right. "What did you say?" I asked.

She said, "Is it a private or public pool?"

I thought to myself, *What kind of question is that?!* I know my face twisted a little bit with confusion as I answered, "It's a subdivision pool, so I guess both?"

She said, "Fat girls don't swim in public pools, but thanks for the invite."

Talk about a self-pity check on my end! I felt so bad for her. I had never once seen this beautiful woman I called my friend as "fat." I didn't know what to say, and before I knew it, the words "At least your fat is distributed evenly" came out of my mouth. *Wait... DID I REALLY JUST SAY THAT?*

Why in the world would I provide an opportunity for anyone to question me about my secret? I will tell you why. My heart broke the moment those words came out of her mouth, because even though she was playing it off as a joke, I could tell she was insecure about the fact that she was overweight. I didn't want her to feel that way, so I decided to share my secret with her right then and there.

I took a deep breath and pulled my skirt up. We both stood there for a few seconds in silence, and then, all of a sudden, she burst out laughing hysterically! Why was she laughing at me? Immediately, my first thought was she was laughing at me because of how my leg looked, so I said, "What is so funny?" I was confused and scared. I laughed nervously with her.

Between each breath she was desperately trying to take, she said, "I thought you wore skirts and dresses because you were Pentecostal!" I began to belly-laugh with her until we were both in tears. We were laughing because of how wrong she was.

Fast-forward to years later, when one evening I told this story to my husband. He helped me realize that I felt she was completely wrong about how people viewed her. He encouraged me and helped me think maybe I was completely wrong about how people viewed me! I really didn't think she was fat, but she did. He helped me understand that my world revolved around me hiding my leg.

This led to a question: What would happen if I stopped hiding it? Maybe not everyone who saw my leg would make fun of me. What if I started a trend of others accepting their bodies and exercising their right to be comfortable in their own skin? What if being brave and vulnerable would help empower others? These questions really got me thinking, but I kept going back to another one: Why me?

No matter how hard I tried to change the answer to that question, the answer stayed the same: Why *not* me? I had this thing attached to my body for a reason. It was part of my identity. I knew I had a purpose in life but didn't know what it was. After that night, I was determined to figure it out because I knew it involved helping others. Little did I know my disability was the key to unlocking my superpower. That was the day I officially "dropped my skirt" and stopped hiding my leg.

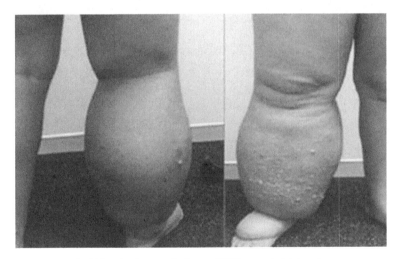

In this photograph from 2013, my right leg is
nearly 200% larger than my left leg.

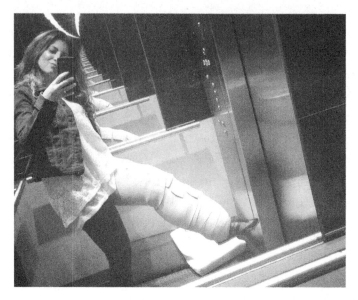

Wearing my wraps with pants for the first time, 2014.

CHAPTER 4:

Shattered Dreams

As I sat at my desk, replaying the conversation with my coworker over and over in my head, I realized I had to help myself if I wanted to help other people with disabilities. That meant I had to find out what was wrong with me and how to fix it. I decided that "it's just swelling" wasn't a good enough answer, and I didn't even want to hear, "It was the way your mother carried you during pregnancy." I was tired of being pushed to the side by doctors who simply didn't have an answer. Technology has changed healthcare in the past thirty years. I was thirty-two years old, and it was about time I got answers.

I decided to Google phrases like "big legs," "elephant legs," and "swollen legs," trying to find something recognizable. The first thing that popped up was literally a picture of elephant feet. As my eyes continued to search, I saw something that really caught my attention: a picture that wasn't a picture of a literal elephant foot. A human leg. I was looking at a man from South Africa whose leg looked just like mine!

You couldn't have peeled me away from the computer screen if your life depended on it! I spent most of my day looking at legs of people in India, South Africa, Algeria, and Thailand. How could this be? I didn't have filariasis, a parasitic disease caused by microscopic worms. I was born this way, so there had to be a better answer.

I continued to search and wasn't going to give up until I found an answer. A fire was lit in me that I hadn't felt in years, and I wasn't about to quit my quest just because a clear answer hadn't presented itself right away.

Then I noticed something that said, "Is elephantiasis curable?" It was the first thing I had found that actually talked about any kind of treatment for those with a leg that looked like mine. I instantly became curious. I kept researching for hours to try to learn more. Eventually I stumbled across a treatment protocol for elephantiasis. The recommended treatment was bandaging the affected limb. I said to myself, "Could I have been bandaging my leg to help reduce its size all these years?"

As I continued my research, I learned about the World Health Organization. I had clicked a link that took me directly to a page on their website, where I read about the lymphatic system. I understood it as an important filtering component to our immune system. I learned that if your lymphatic system malfunctions, fluid can build up in your limbs, causing them to swell. When this happens, you are considered to have a condition called lymphedema. Now we were getting somewhere! I felt like I was getting closer to some answers about what was wrong with me. After reading through their entire website, I saw a link called "Countries." This led me to a doctor in France: Dr. Corinne Becker. I immediately emailed the clinic and said, "I think I may have lymphedema."

The next day, I received a response with a Skype number and time to talk with Dr. Becker. "It appears to be lymphedema" is the only thing I remember from this conversation. As relieved as I was, I was heartbroken. I couldn't go to France for an extended period of time and leave my family here. I definitely couldn't afford it. As I was getting ready to end the call and thank her for her time, she said, "There are doctors in the U.S., but you should come here." I felt time stop for a moment as I sat there in complete shock. There are doctors in the U.S.? How come I had never heard of them?

She was kind enough to give me a few names to look up. I couldn't get off that call fast enough! The first call I made was to my mother. As I was telling her about my recent discovery, she told me that some certified nursing assistant had mentioned that possibility to her years ago, but the doctors dismissed it because my mother hadn't traveled anywhere outside the United States where she could have picked up the parasite while she was pregnant. *WHAT?!* I was beyond upset. Here, all this time, I had been trying to figure out what the heck was going on with me, and my mother had also been dismissed when I was born. How could this be?

I found myself staring at the computer screen in disbelief as I researched the doctors Dr. Becker mentioned during our call. One of them, Dr. Massey, turned out to be a doctor not far from me at all who specialized in lymphedema. How did I not know there was a doctor in Chicago? I could drive to Chicago in a few hours!

After learning this, I contemplated calling Dr. Massey right away. I wasn't sure how I would feel if she told me there was nothing she could do, but I made the call anyway. I was so nervous that I had to redial the phone number twice because I kept hitting the wrong numbers. I didn't know what to expect or what I was going to say when someone picked up. The phone rang three times, and I was getting ready to hang up when the receptionist answered with the name of the office, followed by, "How may I help you today?"

I didn't know how to answer other than, "I think I have lymphedema." She asked me a series of questions and requested I send some pictures in. That evening, I went home and submitted the questionnaire and pictures as requested. I was thrilled to find out I could get in to see this doctor soon.

The next day, I worked things out at my job so I could fly to Chicago to hopefully get a diagnosis. The entire flight to Chicago was a blur. It didn't feel real! I had waited more than 30 years for this moment. Once I landed, I ran to the exit and hopped into a cab. As we pulled up to this beautiful building that stood tall in the middle of Chicago, I stepped out of the cab. I had to take a moment to prepare myself to hear what I had always heard: "It is just swelling."

As I was going to the doctor's office on the fifth floor, I hoped this appointment would be different than all the previous ones. As I got closer, the fear and doubt started to fill my head. I was prepared to leave the doctor's office heartbroken with the words, "Sorry, there isn't anything we can do." The elevator door opened, and I walked down the hall, reading the names on the office doors until I reached Dr. Massey's door. I took a deep breath and walked in.

I walked into this peaceful office that looked nothing like a doctor's office. I was instantly calm. After I signed my life away in a packet full of documents, I was taken into the examination room and asked to remove my skirt and put the sheet on. I tried to pose my hands a certain way so the doctor couldn't see them tremble as my heart pounded in my chest. I knew the doctor was going to move the sheet over so she could get a better view of my leg.

"Can you remove the sheet and stand against the wall so I can take a few pictures before we measure you?" she asked.

I wanted to get up and walk out. I wanted to say no, but I promptly said "Okay," as if I was used to this sort of thing. I don't even know why I didn't want her to see my leg. It was just my fall-back gut reaction when I thought about someone looking at my leg. I didn't want anyone to see this ugly thing attached to me.

She examined me and took measurements of my legs, my range of motion, and the distance between my legs. She then examined my neck and breast area, where lymph nodes are clustered. I lay on the table as she crossed each leg over the other to see at what point it hurt. As I was being examined, I tried to recall if I had ever had such a comprehensive exam at any of my previous doctor appointments. Normally, they would come into the room with their head down, looking at my chart, saying, "What can we do for you today?" then slightly look up at me, then back down to the chart. As I would explain why I was there, they would go over to the computer and type as I spoke. Not once did they listen to me, look at me as I spoke, or acknowledge what I said. This appointment was very different.

I knew I had to be brave. Sometimes when you display courage, deep down inside, you're actually afraid. I felt like I was going to have a panic attack. I was so nervous that my voice quivered when I answered the doctor's questions. I felt sick to my stomach. At one point, I asked if I could sit down because I felt as if I was going to pass out. I had to put my guard down and let this doctor do her job. I had to be vulnerable. Being vulnerable was all that was left between me and finally getting a diagnosis.

The doctor told me I had stage 3 primary lymphedema—Milroy disease, to be exact. Milroy disease is a rare disorder that prevents the lymphatic system from working properly. To receive an actual diagnosis, I needed to complete a test called lymphoscintigraphy. This test is used to map out your lymphatic system with a special dye that is injected between your fingers and toes. Once the dye is injected, you lie on a table and have a series of MRI scans. Wherever the fluid stops is where the obstruction is. This test was the standard test in 2013. Today, another test is offered as well: indocyanine green (ICG) lymphography. The ICG is a green dye that is injected under the skin. You can see real-time movement with a special infrared camera that slides across your limb. These tests are both used for diagnosis.

Every healthy person has a lymphatic system. I discovered I had been born with an incomplete lymphatic system, so it was extremely important for me to understand what happens when it malfunctions. The lymphatic system mimics a sewer system. It removes toxins from your body. It transports fluids and immune cells throughout the body so you can then excrete the toxins through sweat and urination. If your system is compromised or missing, the fluid will accumulate, causing swelling, which is called lymphedema. My lymphedema was considered "primary" because it was present or onset at birth.

That means you can develop lymphedema without ever traveling to a foreign country and exposing yourself to nasty parasitic worms! It was nice to know I wasn't crazy. I knew I hadn't been exposed to anything like that, but it was such a relief to have a clear answer.

According to research, the *FLT4* gene is supposed to produce a protein called vascular endothelial growth factor receptor 3 (VEGFR-3), which regulates the lymphatic system. A mutation such as this causes lymphatic vessels to develop prematurely or not at all, causing lymphedema.[2] In lay-person's terms, your plumbing is backed up. If left untreated, it can cause permanent disability, disfigurement, and possibly death.

Learning about this incurable disease and a possible death sentence if I didn't start treatment right away left me speechless. Mind-numbing shock and fear descended on me upon hearing this diagnosis. I started questioning my grandparents about their parents and their grandparents. I needed to find out who else had this disease in my family. How many generations had it? Was it more prominent on the female or male side? I have since learned that the

---

2   "Milroy disease," *MedlinePlus*, last updated August 18, 2020, https://medlineplus.gov/genetics/condition/milroy-disease/.

disease runs on my maternal grandmother's side of the family. As a matter of fact, my grandmother has recently developed signs of lymphedema in both of her legs.

After 30 years, I had finally found my place in the world as one of 10 million other Americans who suffer from a form of lymphatic disease. I couldn't understand why I felt alone if there were millions of us. Why hadn't the other doctors seen this? Why did they tell my parents it was the way my mother carried me? As the questions kept coming, my frustration kept building and eventually turned into a challenge I felt compelled to take on. I was determined to get more answers.

I still remember my first conversation with my lymphedema doctor. It played a significant role in my new journey toward a healthier life. She was gentle but honest with me. "Your life is going to change, and I can help you. If you don't get this under control, it could lead to death. There is a surgery that can help your disease, and I think you should have it as soon as possible."

I had known there had to be something I could do to take care of my leg, and I hadn't given up until I figured out what that was. After finally finding what I had been looking for, I was simultaneously being told I would need to fight for my life. I was ready. I couldn't die—I had a life to live now that I knew how to live it!

In addition to being told about the life-saving surgery I should have, they also introduced me to techniques to manage the symptoms. My doctor told me about surgical options that could help maintain the disease, and the occupational therapist showed me how to properly bandage my leg.

One of the treatments for lymphedema patients is to wear special bandages called short-stretch bandages. Short-stretch bandages are woven with cotton fibers that provide more resistance and less flexibility than the more elastic bandages you can find at your local drug store. The bandages provide resistance when you move, stimulating the lymph vessels and helping them remove fluid out of the affected limb or body part. For this treatment to be effective, you must have your leg wrapped 24/7 and remove the bandages only to shower.

The potentially life-saving surgery the doctor was referring to is one of the most sophisticated forms of microsurgical lymphatic reconstruction but is under-reseached in the medical field. The unhealthy areas of someone's lymphatic system are reconstructed using healthy lymphatic tissue, including lymph nodes transferred from healthy areas of the body. Both arterial and venous blood vessels are reconnected using an intraoperative microscope to ensure the node transfer survives in the unhealthy area it is being transferred to. Basically, the goal is to create new pathways for the lymph fluid. The surgery is called vascularized lymph node transfer, or VLNT.

In addition to learning about my condition and its treatments, I've learned there are different categories of primary lymphedema; I was diagnosed with Milroy disease (hereditary lymphedema type IA), which is genetically inherited. This is a mutation in the *FLT4* gene, causing vascular issues with my lymphatic system. There is a 50 percent chance of passing this gene to my children for each pregnancy, regardless of the sex of the child. Like so many other parents, I had no idea my children could possibly inherit the same condition.

My daughter, Jade, was diagnosed with a similar but unique lymphatic disorder called lipolymphedema in 2018. I had noticed Jade's body shape was different than most girls her age but never thought about lymphedema. Her symptoms didn't resemble mine. Jade's lower body was much larger than her upper body in certain areas, such as her legs and ankles. Her legs look like tubular columns with little lumps under the skin. Those lumps are fatty deposits, called lipedema, that look like beads. Although the cause of lipedema is unknown, there's research showing hereditary influences. As I get older, I see signs of lipedema in my own body (my thighs and behind), and seeing the same in Jade's body is a telltale sign that lipedema is another factor my family has to be aware of.

Like me, Jade is in chronic pain 24/7. I didn't know she had lipolymphedema until Washington University diagnosed her. This inherited condition is distinguished by the bilateral enlargement of limbs. Basically, the fat cells grow uncontrollably in her thighs, arms, hips, and buttocks. The pressure of the fatty tissue on the lymphatic system causes secondary lymphedema. There are four stages of lipedema and no cure. The treatment plan mimics the lymphedema treatment. My daughter will have to wear compression the rest of her life. I'm thankful for what I went through so I can guide her through this lifelong reduction journey. Luckily, my son is now eight and does not show any symptoms or signs of lymphedema.

This was a lot to take in all at once, but I soaked up as much as I possibly could. After being in the dark for more than 30 years, I felt like a huge weight had been lifted. This disease no longer controlled my life now that I had found hope. I really felt like there was light at the end of the tunnel.

As I flew back home to St. Louis, the surgery weighed heavily on my mind, but my mind was made up before I left the doctor's office. I was going to go through with it, but what really troubled me was the logistics of it all. How would I afford it? Traveling could be challenging with my leg, and I would have to schedule time off work. I also had to consider the costs of the presurgical testing, and of course, being away from my family was going to be tricky.

Still, I was excited to share the news with everyone when I finally made it back home. When I attempted to explain what the doctor said, I became tongue-tied and a bit overwhelmed, so all I could say was, "I HAVE LYMPHEDEMA, AND THERE ARE OTHERS WHO HAVE IT TOO!"

After I was able to explain to my friends, coworkers, and family what lymphedema was, I went into the details of the surgery. I explained about the lymphoscintigraphy test and how I needed that done first to see if I was a candidate for the procedure.

I don't think my mother blinked once as I explained everything. After I was finished, I asked everyone what they thought. The only question that my mother had was what would happen if I wasn't a candidate for surgery. Honestly, I didn't ask nor even think about that being a factor. I couldn't bring myself to think about that. My future was riding on this test. I am the type of person who, once I know the plan, executes one step at a time, and getting the test was the first step.

Three weeks later, I flew back to Chicago to have the lympho-scintigraphy. I never gave any thought during my travels to not being a candidate for this surgery. For some reason, I just knew I would be. Once I arrived, it wasn't long before the testing began. The doctor first injected my hands, then moved to my feet. Because of the thickness of skin between my toes on my right leg (where the lymphedema is), I had to be reinjected a few times due to the needle not being able to penetrate my skin. It was extremely painful. I wanted to kick someone with my so-called "strong leg" every time they injected me. The needle was pretty bad, but it didn't prepare me for how bad the dye would burn as it slowly moved through my body, followed by cramping in my fingers and toes. I was sweating from the horrific pain.

A few hours after the ink injection, a special camera took a series of images as the dye traveled through me, allowing the doctor to see my entire lymphatic system and where the obstruction was. I lay on that table with tears running down my face as I repeated the words "life or death" over and over to myself. If I hadn't kept saying those words, I would have given up. I almost said, "I'm okay with my life," and walked out of the hospital. I really don't know if I would be here today sharing my story if I had given up.

The days that went by as I waited for the test results felt like the longest days of my life. I had the test on a Friday, and the doctor would be out of the office the following Monday! Tuesday couldn't come fast enough, and I really didn't know if I'd even hear from the doctor then! The anticipation of learning the results was intense. I was waiting on information that could change my entire future.

The results came in, and the doctor called me to discuss the next steps. Though I had a calm confidence that I was a candidate for the surgery, I was still relieved to hear the doctor tell me that I was. Not only was I a candidate, but I found out that I was incredibly healthy and had extra lymph nodes in other areas of my body, which made me a great candidate!

The doctor wouldn't move forward with my procedure unless I got a cardiologist, vein specialist, and primary care provider to agree to be my "helping" doctors when I arrived back home for recovery. The next few months were an uphill battle as I fought hard to get multiple doctors to approve this procedure. I had to get test after test with each of them, and of course, they all had to be in correspondence with one another. I replayed the words "you are a great candidate" over and over in my head as I endured all the bone density tests, pregnancy tests, CAT scans, and blood work. Each of them told me I was an "interesting" patient. I asked myself what that meant. I believe they didn't understand my disease very well at the time, so they simply dismissed it.

I was told so many negative things that probably would have scared others out of having the surgery: that it was experimental, that it wouldn't work, that I could die from the procedure, that it would be best to live my life the best way I could now because I would be permanently in a wheelchair by the age of 35, that I wouldn't ever be back on the runway, that I wouldn't be able to be an active mother, that I could most certainly forget about being athletic again.

As I digested what was said to me, I said to myself, "I will die if I don't try this surgery!" I felt like I was about to lose it all. It was almost impossible to find the strength to fight. I had to tap into a power deep within myself to face the challenge in front of me.

I found the spirit of resilience within me. I was going to die if I didn't get the surgery. I needed to have this surgery for a chance to survive and to make sure my kids still had a mother.

I had to see each of the supporting doctors three times before I finally convinced them to approve the surgery for me. After months of appointments and difficult conversations, the surgery was set for May 29, 2013.

CHAPTER 5:

How I Learned to Be a Solution

I finally realized that winning the pageant years ago wasn't time wasted but rather a lesson to use my beauty in a way that can help others. God may have given me a beautiful face but definitely kept me humbled with my leg. I think I know why my cards were dealt this way. When I tell people what is wrong with my leg, they often say, "But you're so pretty!" Over time, I developed a strategy: Capture their attention and have them listen to my story.

My transformation process started in 2013, shortly before my divorce. It turned out my husband had never stopped cheating on me; he had just gotten good at hiding it. That shook my self-esteem a bit. It most certainly has been a journey of discovery for me, though, with moments when I was on the mountaintop and moments when I felt like I was in a deep valley of despair. Looking back through my journey so far, I can confidently say I have had to walk through several valleys before reaching the mountaintops.

Do you ever feel like you are stuck in a valley? If so, write this down: "Setbacks always come. I have the authority to be resilient and do what needs to be done anyway." People often ask me how I transformed my mind to be so tough, think positive, and stay motivated to not give up. Well, I repeated that phrase to myself. I couldn't allow myself to fail. I knew that I couldn't lose hope. I was going to conquer this disease or die trying!

Of course, I had difficult days with my lymphedema and, to this day, still do. One thing that has helped me continue my fight is so simple yet so powerful: I started talking to myself!

It sounds really silly, but I would talk to myself through tough times and give myself some positive reinforcement. I would reward myself after every little victory. Let me give you an example: Lymphedema causes you to have terrible sugar cravings. It can easily turn into a sugar addiction. Yet excess amounts of sugar are dangerous for a person with lymphedema. A few extra sweet snacks in one day cause my leg to painfully swell. As my leg swells with more toxins, I lose all my energy, feel very sluggish, and the brain fog sets in. Hitting the drive-through and getting something deep fried with high amounts of salt is just as much of a problem for me, and the same goes for "bad" fats and grease.

The effects of fueling a body with poor-quality food are exponentially worse when you don't have a properly functioning lymphatic system. My current husband says it's "almost freakish" how "in tune" with my body I am. I feel sick every time I eat junk food, so I made the choice to live healthy to help conquer my lymphedema. After talking to myself and concluding that if I didn't change the way I ate, then almost everything else I did would be in vain, I knew I had to learn how to eat healthy. But, honestly, managing my lymphedema at times was difficult, and I wanted to give up.

Not only is adhering to a strict diet tough, but extensive amounts of exhausting hands-on care are also needed to manage lymphedema. Manual lymphatic drainage (MLD) is a gentle, unique massage that promotes lymph to drain out of the affected area and into areas that drain properly.

Dry brushing is also a common therapy for lymphedema; it is performed with a dry spa brush with natural bristles and consists of a slow and gentle brushing of the skin near your lymphatic channels, which helps remove toxic buildup on the surface of the skin and promotes lymphatic drainage. Afterward, you take a shower to rinse off the dead skin cells.

In addition to these therapies, I had to unwrap and rewrap my leg several times a day to keep the bandages snug because they would loosen up from pushing the fluid out of my leg.

All this healthy eating, drinking plenty of water, safe exercise, regular therapies, and constant compression could quickly be reversed by eating a single burger with fries and a milkshake, or by taking a break from compression for a few hours—just like that!

I would be proud of myself when I was strong enough to endure the cravings for junk food, and I'd compliment myself every time I didn't give in to those cravings. This gave me the drive to keep going. I then learned how to make healthy foods taste delicious, which made eating clean so much easier! I had to talk to myself quite a bit to stay compliant with my compression treatment for a full day. What an accomplishment! I had stage 3 lymphedema. Keeping what felt like a tree trunk compressed all day was no easy task! Celebrating all these small victories paved the way for my new, healthy lifestyle.

I knew the risks of the surgery, and that gave me severe anxiety up until the moment I was wheeled into the operating room. I had waited for this moment for so long. I wasn't going to back down now. On May 29, 2013, I had my lymph node transfer surgery.

I wasn't sure what to expect when I would awake from surgery. The surgeon didn't give me many details about how the surgery would help my leg. I did know I shouldn't expect results right away—it would take nearly two years for the nodes to grow and work on their own before I would see a significant change in my leg.

Initially, the surgery reduced the circumference of my right leg by maybe 15 percent, but I think that was primarily due to wrapping my leg in a sleeve, a layer of cotton called Artiflex, thick foam from my foot to my hip, and 13 short-stretch bandages. The foam was used to break up the fibrotic tissue inside my leg and provide an even layer of compression underneath the bandages.

My right leg was still nearly 200 percent larger than my left leg, so I knew I had a long way to go. I understood my leg swelling wasn't going to go away overnight, just as it didn't "blow up" overnight. My leg started swelling the moment I was born and continued to swell for the next 30 years, and I understood it would take several years to get it back down to a "normal" size—if that was even possible. This journey wasn't a sprint but a marathon, and I had to be mentally prepared.

Recovery was hard. I couldn't bend at the waist for several weeks. I needed help going to the bathroom, bathing, getting dressed, changing bandages, and walking. I needed to rely on others, and I didn't like it! I was the one people relied on, not the other way around. I kept telling myself this was part of the marathon, and I needed the help to fully recover.

Yet recovery was still so hard on me. I found myself alone in the house one day, sitting on my couch and crying because I had to use the restroom and I needed help sitting down on the toilet. In desperation, I called my neighbor to help me. We became very close that day, to say the least.

During the next 18 months of recovery, I battled depression due to the lack of things I could do with my leg and the amount of time it was taking to see improvement. I had to be careful not to hurt the lymph node transfer. Staying bandaged was an undertaking. I had to teach my family how to bandage my leg—something I had only learned how to do myself a few months earlier. My right leg had to be wrapped in bandages 23 hours a day. The only time I could remove them was to take a shower. I will be honest, there were times I wanted to give up and say, "Forget it." The physical pain was minimal compared to the psychological pain I endured.

After two months of feeling sorry for myself, I decided it was time to pull myself together. I couldn't allow my children to see me this way anymore. I didn't want to see myself that way anymore, either.

I shifted my focus to helping others find answers; it would help me stay positive as the time passed. Plus, I wanted answers as to why it took me so long to get a diagnosis. Why did the doctor tell my mother my swelling was due to the way she carried me in the womb? Why didn't doctors talk much about the lymphatic system? They should know what that is, right? I mean, for Pete's sake, they know all the other systems in our body, but not one doctor out of all the doctors I had seen over the last 30 years, with all the education they went through to get their degrees, could tell me I had something wrong with my lymphatic system or that I had lymphedema. Why?

Something was wrong with this picture. I wanted to see how many people were out there who struggled with the same issues and had the same questions. How many people were born with it? Did they have children who had it, and if so, when did they develop it? How were their pregnancies? Did they have complications like me?

I couldn't sit back and wait for answers to magically fall into my lap. I'd started a Facebook page called Ninjas Fighting Lymphedema shortly before my surgery in 2013. I was still coming to terms with my diagnosis, and I wasn't sure if the page would get traction; after all, lymphedema is a rare disease. After a few days of being restless in the hospital, I opened the social media app on my phone and read the private messages from people in different states introducing themselves as "lymphedema sufferers." The messages first trickled in a few here and there every week, then daily, and soon hourly.

My first social media post to the page was a picture of my leg before surgery. I figured if someone was searching for answers like I was and came across this picture, they could reach out to me and I could help. I wasn't sure how I was going to help them, but I wanted people to know they were not alone. The Facebook post went from five likes and zero comments to a few hundred likes with several comments within a month. I remember receiving my first international private message; I was blown away! How in the world had this person heard about my measly Facebook page? Who was I to answer them? These questions went through my mind as I sat there staring at my phone, typing what I was going to say back to this person. I was super nervous!

Over time, as the messages continued to come in, I realized the lack of education and awareness wasn't just an issue in the United States; it was an issue worldwide.

The United States was behind some other countries in terms of readily available treatment, but I saw significant setbacks in the lymphatic community overall as I began to research the disease every day. The lymphatic community consists of patients, caregivers, medical professionals, and peers who are either fighting a lymphatic disease of some sort or helping patients with lymphedema. I was becoming obsessed with lymphedema. I wanted to know everything there was to know about the lymphatic system and the disease. My goal was to be an expert in lymphedema.

After a few months of communicating with others via Facebook, I recognized a pattern of the most common issues in the lymphedema community—issues that were discussed in private lymphedema groups, private messages, and telephone conversations. Everyone struggled with the same problems.

The first problem I saw was the disconnect between doctors and patients. Most doctors receive a maximum of 30 minutes of education on the lymphatic system in their medical training. To pour salt on the wound, they only learn what the lymphatic system does, not what happens when it doesn't work properly and not how to handle a case where a person doesn't have a lymphatic system in part of their body, like me!

Lymph nodes are your body's filtering system. They manage fluid levels, react to bacteria, deal with cancer cells and cell products that would result in diseases or disorders, and absorb fats from the intestines. I believe doctors need to learn about the lymphatic system for more than 30 minutes. This undereducation explained why I never received an early diagnosis.

The second issue I saw was the financial burden of our disease. For us to stay healthy, we must manipulate the lymph nodes manually, since they don't drain on their own. Manual lymphatic drainage moves the skin lightly so the small lymph vessels are not flattened. The movements are slow and rhythmic so the vessels open up. To get this massage, we must see a specialized therapist, not a regular massage therapist.

Even though some patients may have health insurance coverage, lymphedema is not as recognized as many other diseases, and often we are left to figure it out ourselves or simply not get the therapy we need because we can't afford it. This affects the patient's quality of life and access to medical care. For example, if a patient can't pay for the compression garments that must be worn 23 hours each day (and that need to be replaced every six to eight months to keep the inflammation down, keep fluid moving, and prevent the progression of the disease), they can develop cellulitis, a bacterial infection of the skin. Each time you have this infection, it damages the lymph system even more and can result in death.

I, too, experience the economic burden, stress, and mental anguish of not having health insurance coverage for care related to my lymphedema, even though I pay for insurance coverage like so many others. I've even received a letter stating the symptoms of my disease are only cosmetic and treatment isn't covered because of its experimental nature, leaving me in a state of negligence that is out of my control. How am I supposed to take care of my health if I can't get the treatment that is suggested by globally recognized lymphedema doctors?

Healthcare is a requirement if I am to even attempt to be able to live a somewhat normal life, but insurance tries everything they can to avoid paying for my healthcare. When a lymphedema sufferer can't afford or access treatment, it can damage the vital organs, increasing the risk of other diseases, infections, nerve damage, immobility, and, in severe cases, death.

The third issue is isolation. The reason I had never met anyone else like me until 2015 was because they were hiding, just like I did. Society makes us feel like freaks—the whispers behind our backs, the stares, and the jokes made to our faces cause us to hide at home, where we feel safe.

I was tired of hiding, and I was certainly tired of crying every time I heard someone else's story. I had to do something about this, but first, I had to change my own situation. I changed my entire outlook on health and wellness. I thought going to the gym was enough, but going to the gym was a waste of time as long as I wasn't focused on what I was putting into my body. I started eating organic foods, drinking more water, and eating out less, and I stopped drinking alcohol altogether. This change didn't happen overnight, and I definitely had a few setbacks here and there, but I can say I beat my worst enemy—myself!

In 2015, I started dating again. It was a terrifying time for me. I wasn't sure how to date anymore or if anyone would date me because of my leg. It wasn't long before I reconnected with a friend. He knew a little bit about my leg from our previous conversations regarding surgery, but he had never seen it.

As things got serious, I became anxious and was waiting for him to call it off, especially after I noticed my leg wasn't getting better, but worse. He didn't leave. Will, now my husband, has been my rock from the moment we began dating.

We patiently waited for my two-year post-op anniversary before we went back to the drawing board. This time, I knew what questions to ask and whom to ask. I had a complete understanding of my disease but was confused about why the surgery didn't work. I did everything I was told to do, yet my leg was slowly swelling again. This was yet another valley to walk through. I was petrified of falling back into depression.

The fear nearly paralyzed me for an entire year, until someone messaged me on Facebook, asking me to come speak at her lymphedema walk. I wasn't aware of a walk for lymphedema, but I was definitely intrigued. After a two-hour phone call, I decided to fly down to Texas and share my lymphedema story in October on behalf of the Lymphatic Education & Research Network (LE&RN), Texas Chapter. I found myself standing at the podium, mesmerized by the people who looked like me. I felt at home. I shared the same story you are reading in this book in a speech titled "You're Not Alone." I wanted everyone present to know that they were no longer alone. Up until this point, I had only spoken with people via social media, phone, and text messages but had never actually met someone in person with lymphedema.

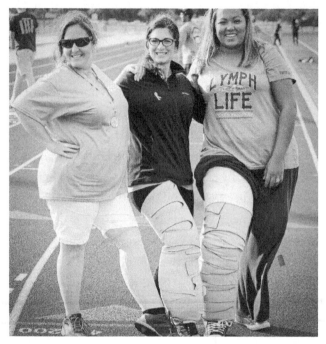

Angelica Flores, me, and a fellow lymphedema thriver (left to right) at the LE&RN lymphedema walk in 2015.

As I headed to the high school track where the walk was being held, I started to see other people who looked like me. I recognized a few faces from my Ninjas Fighting Lymphedema Facebook page and met several more lymphedema patients. One woman walked up to me after I finished speaking and told me she and her family followed me on social media, and when they heard I was speaking, they decided to make a road trip to meet me. *WHAT?!* I couldn't believe that somebody would plan a road trip just to meet me.

When I listened to her story, I felt like I was listening to someone narrate my own story. I fought to keep the tears back when she told me this was the first time she had come out in public with her leg wrapped. She felt compelled to stop hiding and start living with lymphedema after I posted a picture of myself working out with shorts on and my right leg bandaged. This moment made me realize that I was a voice for our lymphatic community. My fear was replaced by courage, and I had a burning desire to speak up for others.

CHAPTER 6:

Advocacy

*W*hen I arrived back home from Texas, I told my husband that I wanted to become more involved with LE&RN. I had seen firsthand how important advocating was, and I wanted to be a part of this movement. He supported me 100 percent.

In January 2016, I became the Missouri Co-Chair for LE&RN. I dove headfirst into finding out everything I could about running an organization. Being a volunteer for a year helped me learn much more than I expected. Within a few months of being the co-chair, I was attending conferences, meeting with lymphatic therapists, and raising money for research, all while working on finding answers I was desperately searching for. At the end of the day, I'm still a patient myself.

In June 2016, I was asked to join LE&RN in California for their annual chapter run/walk. I had never been to Los Angeles and thought this would be a great experience—and it was. The night before the walk, LE&RN hosted a private event for Kathy Bates, and I had the honor to be invited. I kept telling myself to play it cool if I got a chance to speak with her, but honestly, all I could think about was the movie *Fried Green Tomatoes*. I loved that movie!

Kathy had developed lymphedema after a double mastectomy, and this event was being held in her honor for her birthday. Of course, many of her friends and costars from *American Horror Story* came out to support her. I shared my journey with people like Angela Bassett, Sarah Paulson, Frances Conroy, and my all-time favorite, Billy Bob Thornton. Although this was all great, my favorite memory was with someone very special: a young lady named Bri.

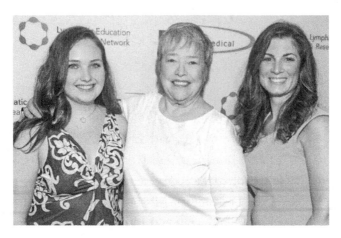

Bri Dobbs, top 2016 fundraiser (left); LE&RN Spokesperson Kathy Bates (center); and me at the 2016 pre-Run/Walk cocktail reception for top fundraisers.

Bri had lymphedema. Bri's mother started following the Ninjas Fighting Lymphedema Facebook page in 2013 in hopes of keeping Bri in a positive mindset. I understood what it was like going through school with lymphedema, and so I had a special place in my heart for this little lady.

When I had found out about the event in Los Angeles, I had reached out to Shellie, Bri's mother. They lived a few hours away, and I was hoping they could make it to the walk. The amount of joy that filled my heart that evening when I saw Bri and her family walk through the door is indescribable. I was in the middle of an interview, and I saw her through the corner of my eye. I politely asked if I could pause for a second, and before the videographer could give me an answer, I was already hugging Bri. You would have thought we had met way before by the way we interacted. This is a common reaction in our lymphatic community. We've experienced loneliness for so long that when we meet someone else with lymphedema, we instantly connect as if we've been in each other's lives for many years.

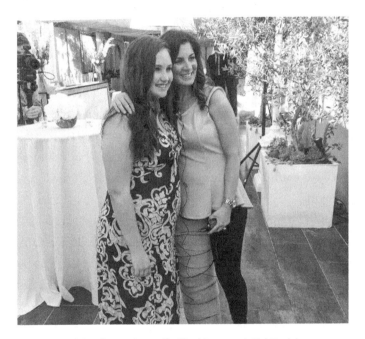

In this photo, I am thrilled to meet Bri Dobbs,
top 2016 fundraiser for LE&RN, at the 2016
pre-Run/Walk cocktail reception for top fundraisers.

We have a unique bond through sharing the experience of living life with lymphedema. This experience defined my desire to help others. I understood what my calling was with lymphedema, and the vision was as clear as the blue sky on a beautiful spring day. As Michael Bloomberg said, "The truth of the matter is: you can create a great legacy, and inspire others, by giving it to philanthropic organizations." I didn't want to give to just any organization; I wanted to create one that reflected strength, perseverance, and of course, a little flare to match my personality. I wanted to create an organization that focused on patients *today*. Research-based organizations are great, and we need to find a cure for lymphedema, but what do we do about the patients who are suffering *now*?

I made the decision to turn the Ninjas Fighting Lymphedema Facebook page into a nonprofit organization in 2017. Anyone who knows me knows that I'm full of life and I love to be challenged, so of course, I wanted an organization that would be in the world's face! I wanted everyone to know who we are, and what we stand for, and to understand that lymphedema is a real disease that wasn't going to stay in the shadows anymore. I wanted to build something I never had: community, a support system, and most of all, a sense of belonging.

If I didn't have the passion I have for others and wasn't as close to the disease myself, I'm not sure I would have it in me to run a nonprofit. I'm not sure I would have been strong enough to persevere through the heartbreaks from constant rejection from people who didn't believe in my vision—not to mention the brick walls politics can create at times regarding adequate insurance coverage.

Luckily for me, I have lymphedema, and it is here to stay, so my passion is also very much here to stay. In my heart, I have a clear definition of who I am destined to be. I'm an inspired philanthropist who wants to leave a legacy of hope.

The Ninjas Fighting Lymphedema Foundation (NFLF) now assists with relieving the financial burdens of out-of-pocket costs related to various forms of treatment, such as garments and therapy. For people who are unsure whether they have lymphedema, NFLF helps find lymphedema doctors to get a proper diagnosis. We promote a positive lifestyle with lymphedema and overall wellness.

NFLF provides a sense of community with other lymphedema sufferers on social media. I take the time to hear their stories because I understand what they are going through. Showing that humanity can still exist is essential to me and is part of the culture of my business. If I show others that I'm no different than them, lead by example, and constantly lift up those around me, then we can build a strong foundation out of love.

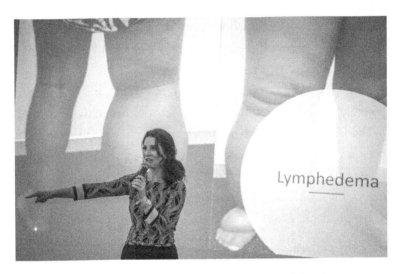

Sharing my story at the 2019 Femme Ascend Conference.

NFLF received 501(c)(3) status in March 2017, and within three years of obtaining our status, the foundation had gained traction all over the world. What started as a local St. Louis nonprofit soon grew across the nation and into a few countries such as Germany, France, Denmark, the United Kingdom, and South Africa. I travel across the United States to share not only my story, but the stories of many other people who suffer from disabilities. I've been blessed to be given the opportunity to share my story all over. I've been interviewed on several news stations and podcasts and for several articles.

As the foundation continued to grow, so did my desire to do more in the community. I wanted to provide more than compression garments. I really wanted to give back to all those who suffer in silence like I did when I was young. I wanted to achieve something greater than great, and I was going to need help. I needed to partner with others who had the same vision.

Andrew Carnegie said, "Teamwork is the ability to work together toward a common vision. The ability to direct individual accomplishments toward organizational objectives. It is the fuel that allows common people to attain uncommon results." And I needed to produce the results I envisioned.

Combine a fantastic team and great timing, and anything is possible! In July 2019, I helped launch the first children's camp in the United States for lymphedema. I was finally able to be that person I never had growing up.

As I continued to fight for the lymphatic community, I was fighting for my health as well. I, too, suffered from the financial setbacks of lymphedema. I couldn't afford to be 100 percent compliant. I was helping others with a very real problem that I suffered from as well.

I had to do more. I decided I wanted to take my voice to the next level and go to Washington, DC, to lobby for our insurance rights! This part is fun for me—I love being the underdog. When I was told insurance doesn't cover our compression garments or surgeries and most of our treatment is an out-of-pocket expense, I was beyond angry. How could this be? Once again, I was on the hunt for answers.

I found an organization called the Lymphedema Advocacy Group, which works to secure passage of the Lymphedema Treatment Act (LTA), a federal bill introduced in the 116th Congress and (as of 2021) waiting to be reintroduced in the current Congress, that will allow coverage of compression supplies by amending the

Medicare statute and improving medical coverage for lymphedema treatment across the board. I signed up right away. This was my chance to share not only my story but the stories of millions of other people who were suffering in silence like I did for so many years.

My first visit to Washington was as nerve-racking as I thought it would be. The first rule of DC is to stand on the right side of the sidewalk and walk on the left, or you will get yelled at or trampled on! I quickly learned that important people have important things to do and, most importantly, places to be. If you stand in the way, you are in their way! I can't tell you how many people walked around me muttering something under their breath about my being in the way. Not that I ever expected to feel like the most important person in the room during these meetings, but I wasn't ready for the big egos.

As I sat in Senator Ron Johnson's office talking about rare diseases and the Orphan Drug Act, I brought up the Lymphedema Treatment Act; I was midsentence when a member of his office said, "Healthcare isn't a human right." As he continued to speak, I started unwrapping my leg, and by the time he finished saying, "It will raise costs and kill jobs," my leg was out in the open and the room was silent.

I looked at him and said, "And you were saying?" I lost all fear and was downright angry. I made sure they saw me as the most important person in that room.

Why is it that we can be fined for not having healthcare coverage, yet I was being told healthcare is a privilege, not a right? As I pointed at my leg, I said, "Medical issues such as lymphedema strip the quality of life away from me in ways that you don't understand. This 'privilege' you like to refer to is being taken for granted by people like you. What privilege am I paying for if I can't get the coverage I need to survive?" I never got an answer, but I sure did get his attention.

I knew I wanted to help people at a young age, hence why I became a nurse. Once that was taken away from me, I thought I would never be able to live a life of giving or serving others. At the time, I was too afraid to help myself and didn't know I had the gift to help others in a different way.

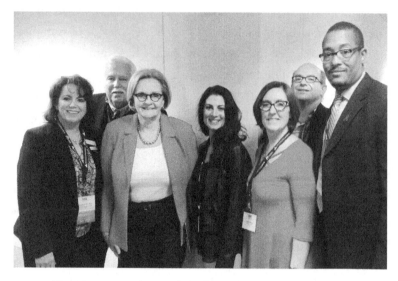

Here I am meeting with U.S. Senator Claire McCaskill (third from left) and members of the National Organization for Rare Disorders (NORD) team in Washington, DC, for Rare Disease Week 2017.

Throughout my journey, I've discovered that I never would have found my purpose in life if I didn't have lymphedema. It's funny how things play out sometimes. My leg is my blessing. The bottom-line intention of the NFLF is to save lives, but as I sit here with a new perspective on my own life, I know being the source of hope for so many others kept me from self-destruction.

I am often asked how I stay so motivated helping others when I have my own set of problems. The real answer is that people like you reading this book have kept me motivated throughout my journey. When I'm on the phone and hear tears flowing on the other end, followed by, "Please help me," or "Thank you for doing what you're doing," I can't help but remain focused. Even when my own life is crumbling at times, I don't let anything get in the way of my mission. I always maintain an "others first" mentality and am determined to make a difference in the world through service. I know I'm not alone in my efforts because I have so much support all around me. If you're reading this book and you have lymphedema, please know you are not alone.

Remember the words of Stephen Hawking, from his 2012 London Paralympic Games Opening Ceremony speech: "We are all different. There is no such thing as a standard or run-of-the-mill human being, but we share the same human spirit."

CHAPTER 7:

Create Your Truth

As the foundation has grown, I've grown with it. I knew I had to fight for my life just as hard as I fight for everyone else's, but if I'm being honest, it is easier to fight for them than for myself. I think it's a coping mechanism for me.

My depression was driving the stress and anxiety of my health condition, leaving me feeling somewhat helpless. During my 18-month recovery from my first surgery in 2013, I focused on the foundation, my health, and my story with lymphedema. I decided I was going to live life to the fullest no matter the outcome.

My efforts gained national attention. People were intrigued by my positive mindset as I started to openly share my journey on social media. Before I knew it, I was asked to share my story with local news stations. At first, I declined the requests. I wasn't ready for that, but after much convincing, I realized that I needed to share "our" story. Several lymphedema patients had the same story as me, but they weren't given the opportunity to share theirs. I had to put on my pageant face and perform. I advocated everywhere I went! If I had an opportunity to educate, I did.

I welcomed the stares I would get in public. Several people were brave enough to ask me what happened. By the time I finished explaining the disease, they would say, "I know someone who has that," or "I didn't know what that was, but I know someone who has to wear the garment." Having the power to educate comes with the responsibility to educate! I was so focused on spreading knowledge, I didn't care if I had to educate the world one conversation at a time.

As I continued to gain exposure, so did my fight with lymphedema. A lymphedema therapist mentioned a doctor in St. Louis who could perform the specific surgery I needed, called suction-assisted protein lipectomy (SAPL). The SAPL surgery is for late-stage lymphedema patients like me. "Late-stage" means the lymphedema has progressed to such an extent that the fluid has turned into a solid and will continue to grow until it is surgically removed. The SAPL surgery was supposed to remove the solid buildup permanently.

My journey thus far had taught me to remain humble and that it's okay to struggle, it's okay to cry, and to always practice kindness, patience, and empathy. The first surgery was initially successful, but the nodes soon died from fluid overload. My filtering system was clogged again, and my leg was back to the point of not responding to MLD therapy, which I had to have done three times a week, to no avail. Nothing was moving, or if it was, it was very little.

My leg was full of solids that had accumulated over the years from my chronic lymphedema. The solids (abnormal accumulation of protein-rich fluids that turn into fatty deposits) are permanent and cannot effectively be treated with therapy. As I mentioned earlier, once you reach this stage, the only thing left is surgery. We were finally getting somewhere! And like that, I was set for the operation after my consultation.

In December 2016, I had the SAPL surgery. As I woke up in the recovery room, I noticed my leg was smaller, but I wasn't sure how much smaller it was until I fully came to. My heart sank when I uncovered my leg. It was a lot smaller, but not what I had expected.

The doctor had done his best, but I was too severe of a case. Maybe I was meant to have this leg after all.

Later that night, as I was in and out of consciousness from the pain medicine, I had the same recurring dream of walking in the park with shorts on. As I came to, I said, "My fight isn't over." I wasn't even out of the hospital before I began to plan my third surgery. I wasn't going to give up. I couldn't; too many people were depending on me, including myself.

I found myself circling back to a certain doctor every time I would research the surgery. I knew this doctor but avoided him because I never thought I would be able to afford him. I knew he was the best, but for some reason, I didn't think I deserved the best; otherwise, I would have found a way a long time ago.

A year later, I flew to California and met with him: Dr. Jay Granzow. I couldn't believe it! I was here! I didn't know how I was going to pay for it, how I would manage to be away from my kids for several weeks, or even where I was going to stay, but the one thing I did know was that I deserved this and I was going to find a way.

When I walked into his office, he smiled gently and said, "I'm happy you're here." He and I spoke on several occasions, and he told me from the first conversation that he could help me. He could have said, "I told you to come to me from the start," or "Why did it take you so long?" but he didn't. He knew why it took me so long and didn't need to remind me. I was much calmer showing my leg this time; I had become good at it by this point. I now used my leg as a visual for everyone so they understood what untreated lymphedema looks like.

After the consultation, we had to submit the procedure to the insurance company for approval. I had no worries. The first two were approved with zero issues. Several months later, we received the first letter of authorization. I was jumping up and down, even with an extra 30 pounds on one side! You couldn't take the smile off my face!

Then the hammer came down. Right as I was planning for the surgery, another letter came from my insurance company, stating the first surgery I had in St. Louis was an error, and this surgery would not be approved because there was an exclusive change to my policy stating no coverage for lymphedema or treatments.

I was in Washington, DC, lobbying for the Lymphedema Treatment Act when I received the news. I had started the process two years earlier, in 2016, right after my failed SAPL procedure, and *now* this was their response?

I was not just upset; I was empowered by rage. If this could happen to me, it could happen to those who don't have a voice. My fight was no longer about me; it was about our community, and what better place could I have been than on Capitol Hill? I took that letter with me to every representative, senator, and anyone else who would listen. After getting a few senators and representatives behind me, I dug further into this issue. I finally found out what happened.

The insurance coverage I had was through my previous employer, whom my husband at the time was working for, and they were self-insured, meaning rather than paying an insurance company to pay the claims, the employer reviewed the claims and—if they saw fit—would pay the claims through a third-party administrator. The insurance company told me this employer was the one making all the decisions on my claim, and I would have to take my appeal to them.

What does that even mean? How does my employer make the calls? I had been with this company for 10 years, and they had been supportive at first, until I wasn't released to return to work until my health showed improvement. Even though I was no longer employed with them, my husband still was. They were upset that I hadn't been able to return to work, so they didn't want to pay for the procedures.

The company could decline appeals with reason. The problem was, they didn't have a valid reason. It took two appeal requests to figure out their "reason" for denying coverage for my surgery. An unqualified physician (a podiatrist) who had zero lymphedema knowledge was the medical professional denying my procedure. After we discovered that, we requested the files they kept on my case, but they only provided some and refused to release all of them.

We decided to open a federal review case as a last resort if this last appeal was denied. In the review, we were going to point out not only the insurance company's actions, but the employer's as well, if they would not change their decision. I sent a letter to the insurance company as well as to the employer and my state senator and representative. In this letter, I outlined the ailments of lymphedema, the rigorous, constant treatments it necessitates, and that my insurance refused to cover lymphedema-related supplies, treatments, or procedures. I explained how difficult this time-consuming medical maintenance made full-time employment and pointed out the lack of understanding of the condition among employers.

I explained that my health insurance company considered lymphedema a "cosmetic" condition rather than a medical condition, despite its life-threatening effects. I explained that each lymphedema specialist I had consulted recommended surgery. I shared the timeline of my requests and appeals for coverage and how I was not even allowed to receive a full explanation of why the procedure was being denied, and that it was being denied by a doctor who had no experience with lymphedema. I concluded with the promise that "I will continue to advocate for patients like myself" and the reminder that "We have the RIGHT to coverage (especially when we pay for it)."

It's also important to note that my employer should not have been in charge of reviewing my case. I had received harsh treatment right before I went on medical leave in 2016. For example, I had to talk to the HR director about my time off, and when I returned to my desk, a colleague threw a box at me and said, "I'm so sick of you and your disease," because she didn't want to take over part of my job while I was gone. Who acts like that in a professional setting?

Then the text messages started coming from coworkers telling me that I needed to work from home while I was recovering from SAPL. It appeared the HR director was sharing my health information with other people and giving her own opinions about why I wasn't released to work yet.

Then the marketing director made a false claim on LinkedIn that I was taking money from the Ninjas Fighting Lymphedema Foundation to live on, which was simply not true. We hadn't even received a single donation yet! That's how new our status was at the time.

I couldn't understand why my coworkers were treating me this way. I didn't leave the company to work for another company; I was trying to gain my health back so I could work again! I took these findings to my former boss and told him this was slander and it needed to be addressed. Soon after, I received a LinkedIn message stating this outrageous accusation had been removed. I could go on and on, but you get the idea. Frankly, even if I would have been cleared to return to work, I never would have gone back to that toxic environment. The fact is, I didn't get the medical release to go back to work until all my surgeries were completed and I was fully healed.

Because they didn't like the fact that they would have to pay for my surgery again when I wasn't even working there, the office thought they could walk all over me and pull these scare tactics on me and my husband. It was completely unprofessional, wrong, and downright low how my former employer treated me during this trying time.

While I was at home recovering from the SAPL and working on the next set of appeals, the harassment continued. The CEO of the company called my husband's office and said he would sue us for the very little we had if we didn't remove a post on social media I had made about how unhappy I was that my former employer was giving me such a hard time, which he considered slander. They tried to say that they never changed my insurance coverage nor would they decline my coverage, despite the email I had from the insurance company stating otherwise.

What he failed to realize was that I had months of documentation of being harassed and bullied for my fruitless requests to file complaints on multiple occasions. At this point, I was angry and tired of this company controlling me even after I was gone. Just because this corporation could get away with it in most cases didn't mean I was going to let them rob me of my chance to improve my quality of life. This wasn't only about me anymore; it was about the entire disabled community. I was tired of being treated like this, and I had a fire in me to fight for all of us.

Bullying happens primarily in private settings and normally by a person in authority, and they often don't leave material evidence. Don't ever think it happens "by accident" either; it is a deliberate action, often planned out. After a decade of this, I was ready for a battle. What I was about to do had never been done, and I knew my plan could backfire on me, but I couldn't back down. I said,

"Nobody will tell me what my quality of life will or will not be," and showed my cards.

I sent a 16-page letter to the appeals department stating what the company was doing was unethical and cited the Americans with Disabilities Act. I decided to send copies of the complaints I'd requested to be filed, harassing text messages, emails, and voicemails. I sent this letter to the CEO, executive vice president, HR director, and most of the corporate office. I also made sure their attorney, the insurance company, and insurance department got a copy of the letter. The gloves were off at this point, and I wasn't holding back.

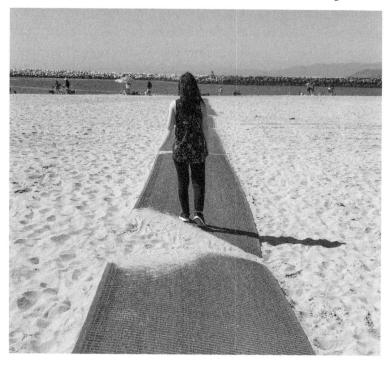

My first time walking without assistance after the SAPL in 2018.

Two weeks later, I received another letter stating, "After careful review, we have decided to approve your procedure." *I beat the bullies at their own game!* I was tired of being suppressed, and I wasn't going to be bullied anymore. Having a disability is hard enough on our daily lives without adding toxicity at the workplace. On September 23, 2018, my dream came true. I had the surgery!

This fight wasn't a sprint; it was a marathon, and I had no idea what to expect next. It reminded me of Marla Runyan, the first legally blind runner to compete in the Olympics. I couldn't see the path in front of me, but I knew I could win if I followed my instincts and kept going.

CHAPTER 8:

Invisible Disability

As I came out of the anesthesia, I remember looking around to find my husband's face. I wanted to see his reaction before I pulled the covers back. I wasn't sure if I could handle another failed surgery, so I was pretty nervous about pulling the covers off. I also had a moment where I didn't know how I would feel not having my big leg anymore. You see, my big leg had been my identity for my whole life, yet I wanted it gone for obvious reasons.

I identified myself with lymphedema to the point of almost becoming prideful of having it. Not that that is a good thing, but it's how I dealt with it. I owned it with everything I had. I had shifted my thinking to build a special kind of resilience, and now I wasn't going to stop until I changed the public view of "disability." I think I developed this pride to protect my self-esteem against the negative stigma that comes with disability, but what would I hide from now if I no longer *looked* disabled? Many disabilities are invisible to others at first glance. I know some people identify with them like I do; however, there are others who hide their disabilities to avoid discrimination, like I did for so long.

Once I was in my room and settled, my husband came in with a massive smile on his face. He told me everything the doctor had told him, but it was all a blur to me. The next morning, the therapist came in to unwrap my leg and get me up and walking. As she pulled the covers back, I saw several bandages that went all the way up my leg. I had all this foam and wrapping on my leg as if I still had a large limb. As she slowly removed each bandage, I took a deep breath, not because of the physical pain but because I was preparing myself for emotional distress if the surgery was a failure.

I couldn't believe my eyes. For the first time in my life, I had a knee—and an ankle! I had been in the elephantiasis stage (a condition characterized by gross enlargement of an area of the body, especially the limbs), and the dorsum of my foot was covered by an extra flap of skin and squared off underneath. I hadn't been able to see my ankle for years!

Tears fell down my face. I couldn't feel them much from all the pain medication, but I felt the wetness on my cheeks. Shortly after that, the doctor came to check on me. They had removed 16 inches of skin and four liters of mostly solid, fatty tissue. I literally lost 30 pounds overnight!

The initial recovery was long and painful—so painful that I questioned why I did it at first. As the days grew into weeks and the weeks grew into months, the pain subsided, and I was able to focus on a new life. I had to relearn how to walk, but it was worth it because, finally, for the first time in my life, I was able to live a normal life.

Living a "normal" life was hard for me to understand. I noticed that when I went out in public, nobody stared at me anymore. People didn't stop to ask me what happened to my leg. If they did, it was because they had either seen me on the news or read an article about me. It was so weird to me that I was having normal conversations with people. I wasn't talking to them about what they saw in my physical appearance. I was confused about how to feel about this.

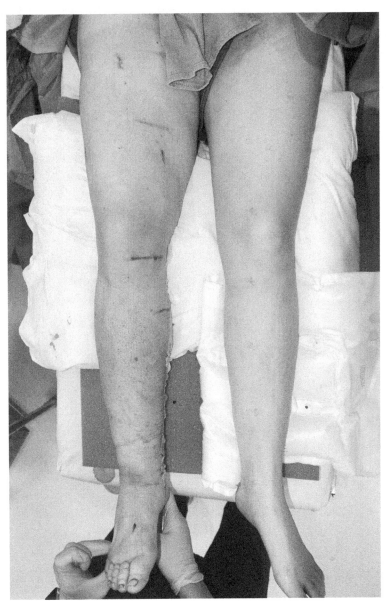

My legs postsurgery in the operating room, 2018.

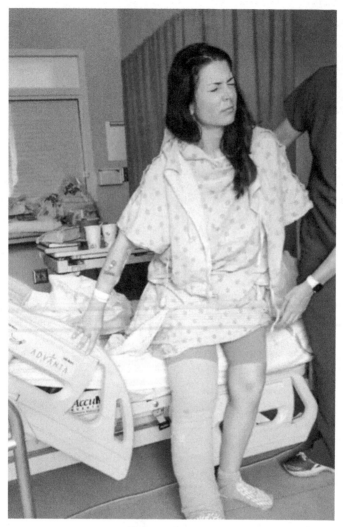

My first time standing up after the 2018 SAPL surgery.

I still have the disease and always will—unless, of course, a cure is found. The surgery was one tool in my treatment plan, a tool that would allow me to live life without pain. You can't cure or fix something that isn't there (lymph nodes), but I could at least get the lymphedema to a manageable stage. I still see a therapist for MLD;

wrap on occasion, such as in the evening or when it is blistering hot outside; and I monitor ALL of my food. For as long as I live with lymphedema, I will always be considered disabled. However, it isn't as visible anymore.

Who is the beauty queen with the big leg now if she doesn't have a big leg anymore? I began to understand other disabilities besides lymphedema. I saw the reality of invisible disabilities. I was now defending mine as much as treating it. Nobody should ever be attacked for their disabilities, visible or not.

The fact that people have to defend their medical conditions doesn't sit well with me. I'm sure it doesn't sit well with anyone else who has an invisible disability, either. I have been on both sides of disability: the visible and invisible. Neither side is easier than the other. They are both equally difficult to deal with, but I believe, in many cases, being disabled can be what you make of it. My lymphedema is my blessing, and I wouldn't ask for anything to be different. I would not be the person I am today if I hadn't experienced the things I experienced.

Today, I'm the mother, the athlete, and the model I knew I could be. Most importantly, I found my voice through my valleys and now understand that my disability is my superpower.

My name is Amy Rivera, and I dropped my skirt to spread hope in a world that desperately needs it.

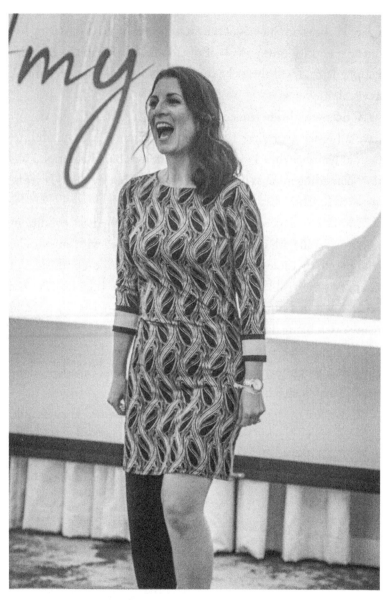

On stage at the 2019 Femme Ascend Conference.

Lymphedema Resources

The Lymphedema Treatment Act

To learn more about the Lymphedema Treatment Act (LTA), a federal bill that aims to improve insurance coverage for lymphedema treatment by amending the Medicare statute to allow coverage for compression supplies, visit lymphedematreatmentact.org.

Dr. Jay Granzow

If you are suffering from lipedema or lymphedema and need surgical assistance, consider contacting the offices of my surgeon, Dr. Jay Granzow, at lymphedemasurgeon.com.

National Organization for Rare Disorders

The National Organization for Rare Disorders (NORD) is a patient advocacy organization that focuses on rare diseases such as primary lymphedema through programs of advocacy, research, patient services, and education. Learn more at rarediseases.org.

Acknowledgments

I dedicate this book to the lymphatic community for the incredible support they have given me during my personal journey with lymphedema.

I would like to personally thank the three men who stood by me from the beginning:

Fred E. Miller, who passionately taught me how to share my story. His efforts have brought immeasurable self-worth to my awareness.

Larry Cohn, for believing in me from the beginning. Larry's positive impact will remain in my heart as long as I live.

Will Rivera, my husband, who has loved me through this entire self-healing journey. Will has brought out the BEST version of me by helping me understand my gift: my lymphedema.

Thank you, family, friends, and supporters for not giving up on me. I will always remain grateful for your love, trust, and honor. Because of you, I won my fight.

About the Author

Amy Rivera believes living a purpose-driven life shouldn't be directed by obstacles in our path but rather should align with our values. She left the corporate medical world to pursue her calling and live life through philanthropy.

Amy was born with an incurable disease called lymphedema that left her immensely disfigured. She developed an activist mindset as she feverishly fought to better her own quality of life through medicine, nutrition, fitness, and faith. Against all odds, her journey led her to become one of the few who accomplished the seemingly impossible. She was able to reverse her disease from the worst known severity to being able to manage it with minimal maintenance.

By facing adversity to the highest level of degree with a rare disease, Amy understood what it was like to be alone. She created a community of laughter, life, and education so we can discover how to awaken our inner resilience and take authority over our own lives. Together, we can live, laugh, and learn how to heal.

Made in the USA
Columbia, SC
31 January 2022

55096267R00055